ACKNOWLEDGEMENTS

I am so grateful for the Big Love and support my friends and family have offered me, not just during the course of writing this book, but during the course of what brought it about. In particular, I am grateful to my Hapa family who held me so gently when I fell--that experience taught me a big lesson when it came to knowing in my heart that there really is nothing to fear but fear itself.

I am grateful for every heartfelt conversation I have had along this journey, and the conversations I will have tomorrow. At the risk of leaving someone out, I'm going to let Big Love in, and remind you that all of my loving people know who you are, I might not mention you each by name, you are irreplaceable to me.

Let us always be friends and family.

Chapter 1
Introduction

Just how I Involved Comprehend the Trouble

I've been burning things since I can keep in mind.

Don't get me wrong, I'm not a pyro, I don't shed points like that. I don't man the fire when camping, or the BBQ when food preparation. No, I don't burn items just to enjoy quite shades relocate. I don't wish to ruin points.

I such as to burn other things, as well as I do it truly well.

For a long period of time I indulged in working day and night, as well as the candle at both ends. I melted plenty of calories, and also grams of fat. I melted through level programs as well as details. I've melted up monotonous jobs and a couple of beginning- up business.

Yep. For years at a time I ran too warm, too quickly, up until I just began shedding up from the within out.

There was one considerable event, however, that was like splashing the fire with lighter fluid as well as stoking the flames. I got expecting with my little lady, my first infant at age thirty-five. At regarding 3 months in, my thyroid revved to a hyperactive bonfire. My body immune system ran amuck striking my thyroid and the cells behind my appropriate eye. It turned me into a shivering and weak destroyed covering of an individual. It made my hair fall out and also my skin dry up, it made my lips pale and also my eye lump. I saw dual and also felt insane.

It didn't assist that my eyelids had actually additionally withdrawed and I looked like the stressed out fanatic I felt like on the within. I was in a continuous state of shock and uncertain of everything. With my heart competing to two times its all-natural speed when relaxing, I was burning with years of my life just being awake. I sweated constantly from being as well overheated within, and also I couldn't rest 2 hours right if my life depended on it.

And it did. My life depended on me having the ability to decrease my system adequate to just rest so I might be a parent, a spouse, as well as handle a work as well as my home. I was bewildered, as well as had no concept what was taking place within me. I didn't feel like myself and also I didn't talk about it with any individual.

Gradually, through the course of my pregnancy as well as the first year after it, I watched, enthralled by the fire burning within, as my health and wellness went up in fires.

I keep in mind strongly an occasion that made me realize I had let whatever was taking place reach a critical moment like it was the other day. I was in the washroom at the neighborhood Target on a Saturday as well as it was packed. My hands were trembling. My mama was outside with the cart, waiting. I had my eleven-month- old daughter on the transforming table and I was putting sweat. The hand dryer was appropriate alongside me, regularly pumping out warm air and also noise. Youngsters were shouting and commodes were purging. My little girl was unbelievably client. She really did not cry, she simply looked around.

I didn't like altering her on the plastic drop down table. It looked like she can roll off of it; that the strap was also slim. My hands trembled a lot I battled to click it closed. I kept one hand on her and I attempted to constant myself so I could obtain the wipes, the cream, and the diaper. I was panicking for no noticeable reason apart from I felt so out of control and also jumpy. I tried to maintain my ideas as well as feelings all contained yet there was poop anywhere and I was flipping out because the mother behind me, waiting to utilize the table, was blazing. It felt like it took permanently to end up. Sweat ran off my nose and also melted away my make-up. It ran into my eyes, made it difficult to see. I was so disoriented, but in some way I concentrated and took care of each of the steps. I relied on the strap on the transforming table just enough time to shove everything back into my backpack as well as I made use of both hands to whiz it closed. I drew it over my shoulder and also dealt with the clasp on the table. Lastly I pinched it hard enough and also picked up my lady. My arms were drinking and also I prayed that I wouldn't drop her. Sweat rolled down my back like a river.

Stars filled my vision as well as I leaned against the wall. Females as well as kids hurried past me. I made it to the door and entered the hallway. My mommy was right there as well as I saw the alarmed expression on her face when my leg gave out and also I fell apart to the flooring. I thought, "Do not drop her, do not drop her." It all happened so fast. I got on the floor and searching for. My daughter existed, risk-free, standing in front of me, so solid, protecting me, her little distribute extended, arms flung sideways to protect me, an appearance of deep issue on her smart child face.

My daughter was just about one. I was a postpartum nursing brand-new mom, believing this must be typical, and also yet understanding that something was extremely incorrect with me. It wasn't till I recognized I was having constant migraine headaches as well as my eye was aching, type of changing shape, and my vision ended up being too consistently dual for me to drive, that I started to follow the indicators and also figure out that I had Tomb' Disease. By the time I saw the best medical professional that would suggest medication to a nursing mom, I had thyroid levels that were 7 times normal, and also I had a resting heart rate two times as rapid as it must be. It was wintertime as well as twenty levels outside and also I was sweating in a container top. I could not sleep in the evening, I would simply sweat the bed with visualized concern, as well as I was horribly worn down all of the moment. I had no stamina. Yet the worst component, the outright worst component, was that psychologically as well as psychologically, I was a totally gone nuts weeping mad absent-minded determined mess and my relationship with my hubby, my buddy in the whole world, was under severe but unseen stress. I can not get clear, about anything, as well as I did not believe I would make it through the hell that entraped me.

If you have picked up this book, it is since you or someone you love recognizes specifically what I am discussing, and also my heart goes out to you. It wraps around you in a large hug that claims, "Don't worry, I understand this is rough, however there is comfort and alleviation beyond.".

I frantically wished to hear that when I was in the thick of it.

After one year on thyroid medication and also beta-blockers (and also a host of adverse effects that were virtually as poor as the alleviation), I had a regular monthly visit with my endocrinologist. I can barely jump my little woman on my knee and also yet I asked him how much time he thought I could need to take this medicine as well as be a stranger in my very own skin prior to I went back to normal, prior to I got back to me.

He took a look at me specifically and claimed with gut wrenching pity in his eyes, "Heather, many females never ever come off medicine. Also if you were to radiate your thyroid or surgically remove it, you would be on some sort of thyroid medication forever.".

It seemed like he read out loud my life sentence to imprisonment.

I would certainly never once again be that blissful woman who was so delighted she started and also had a baby with the male she had actually liked for over half her life. Would I ever before recognize the real me again, would certainly my other half? Would certainly my little lady mature with a fanatic for a mommy? Was the me that was well balanced, bright, caring, individual, tranquility, nurturing ... deeply pleased ... gone ... permanently?

The Horror.

" Many females never ever come off of drug. Even if you were to radiate your thyroid or have it gotten rid of, you would certainly get on some type of medicine for the rest of your life. Furthermore, if you don't take steroids for your eye you'll go blind.".

No one intends to listen to these words, however they are claimed all too often to clients that are pleading for some alternative. My customer, we will certainly call her Sparrow, met me at a very susceptible moment in her life. She had actually just been made to hang around in severe concern about her eye. Her eye doctor had her nearly persuaded that if she really did not take steroid therapy for her eye, she would definitely go blind. Deeply worried and also worried due to the fact that her instinct put her up in arms with an expert, she shouldn't have ever needed to picture such a result. When we first spoke as well as agreed to interact, she additionally dedicated to waiting eight weeks to commence any kind of type of steroids. Eight weeks later, she turned up for an appointment with a brand-new doctor, only to locate that her condition had actually supported as well as it had not progressed.

It is incredible how much of an impact the words we hear from people we trust have on us.

One of my innovative readers for this manuscript contributed her thoughts about this:.

" That is such an important point. All of us require to understand this, yet likewise the truth that nobody else yet ourselves has the obligation to secure ourselves from the unfavorable messages around us. That is not to state that we then come to be and also ever suspicious beings, but that we should maintain a sober mind when getting details. And also, trust fund what the digestive tract states regarding it. One a lot of people surrender themselves to the hands and also egos of doctors, most of which are simply drug auto mechanics as opposed to therapists.

This, partially, is not their mistake however instead a stopping working of a system that teaches them to separate the mind, heart and soul, and also aims at administration of a populace instead of assistance of a person.

In Dr. Jeffrey McCombs, DC publication "The Whatever Guide to the

Autoimmune Diet plan," he talks about the power of the placebo impact yet additionally of the nocebo effect (I never ever heard the term up until reviewing this), which is the reverse of placebo impact: "If somebody believes that she will certainly get sick, after that she is most likely to get sick." (p. 83) "Harvard scientist Ted Kaptchuk has actually revealed that when clients are informed to anticipate a certain adverse effects from their treatments, they manifest them. Lisa Rankin, MD, calls this clinical hexing.

In an article in Psychology Today, Dr. Rankin states, 'Whenever your physician tells you have an 'incurable' ailment or that you'll get on drug for the rest of your life or that you have a 5 percent chance of a five-year survival, they're essentially cursing you with a type of 'clinical hexing.' What a person thinks may be as essential a factor in creating autoimmunity as anything else." (p. 84).

The above example is one end of the range, the various other end of the spectrum, the positive and love based, is something I experienced and it made all the difference for me. When I was diagnosed, I just told a few individuals close to me, however somehow the ideal woman heard about it and called me.

She informed me her tale. After her kid was birthed she was detected with Graves' Condition and also after a year on medication, she naturally entered into remission. I clung to that story like my only lifeline. Somebody I recognized had actually done it, and also done it in one year.

Western medicine is amazing in all it has to offer crucial scenarios. I can not have turned this ship around if it hadn't been for PTU. PTU was my thyroid medication of selection. Mix that with beta blockers as well as I had an alcoholic drink solid enough to physically ground me. It checked me out of the physical distress, however it additionally separated me from myself emotionally and also emotionally.

Making peace with Graves' Condition and also Thyroid Eye Condition is difficult since they are vicious conditions that bring upon psychological and also emotional torment. I appreciated the aid the drugs gave me when I required them most, yet long term, I wanted the option because those things were poisoning my spirit. I wanted to maintain my body and soul undamaged, and also just cool down enough to leave medication. Because very same source, Dr. McCombs cited the previous head of study for the pharmaceutical firm GlaxoSmithKline, Allen Roses, MD as having actually specified, "The large majority of medications just work in 30 or half of the people." (p. 79) McCombs goes on to state that medicines are undoubtedly not the final option.

While those medications we turning my physical symptoms around, they also made me seem like a darkness of myself, perpetually boring, a gap.

I was wed to my partner of sixteen years, he was my friend, I had simply had an infant, and life was pitch black. It really did not make good sense.

The physical symptoms misbehaved enough (weakness, trembles, jitters, sweats, weight fluctuations), yet after that there were the complications that made me want to just conceal. I really did not intend to take added medications for those irritable symptoms, as well, or make any type of choices regarding anything, or be social at all. I was angry as well as quick-tempered. Incredibly, I could keep it with each other enough to navigate mothering, however battled when it became a better half, as well as trembled at the thought of mosting likely to a celebration or back to function. I felt worried all the time and also dropped points or run across points generally. I entirely did not have social elegance.

Simply put, I wished to hideout until I improved, yet I seriously doubted whether I would certainly ever improve. I wanted to search in the mirror and see myself. Heck, I intended to see duration. I had such negative double vision I couldn't drive and I can barely utilize the computer or my phone. Life was grinding to a stop and doing the daily points called for by contemporary life was overwhelming. I desired out of discomfort and also off of pills. I wanted support and also simple tool set for improving.

When I first spoke to Sparrow, we invested a hr on the phone with each other just getting to know each various other. I asked her a lot of inquiries regarding where she was appropriate then with every little thing, and what her experience has actually been like thus far. It was full of tests and also adversities, pain and also distress. In the long run, I asked her why she called me. She informed me she went to the end of her choices, which she really did not such as sensation powerless, and at the impulse of her medical professionals' suggestions. Particularly because, based upon her research, she had not been convinced that the remedy they were providing would function long-term.

She needed a tool set, as well.

Having her ophthalmologist impart an anxiety of going blind did nothing to recover Sparrow, or even assist her choose, however her doctor can not recognize why she would certainly have a hostility to radiating the muscles in her eyes. It was the option he recognized of, and also what he might offer her currently.

It was her intestine that informed her it had not been the right choice.

My intestine hasn't been black and also white concerning every one of this. I have significantly taken advantage of drug and 3 eye surgeries, yet likewise identify that the refined body-mind-spirit recovery needs to have a different avenue of approach.

Healing is what happens when we locate an approach we believe in, one we count on, and one we have actually familiarized. Well, when I went to my wits finish, I chose I recognized myself truly well as well as trusted I would discover the technique that functioned based upon what I thought and also recognized to be true. I began to heal from within when I took responsibility for identifying what was mosting likely to function and also what wasn't.

And afterwards I took obligation for doing what benefit the remainder of my life.

This is where it gets hard. It's that long-lasting dedication that typically is the greatest challenge to lasting health, as well as this is where Sparrow stumbled. Like countless other ladies I have talked to, she had actually gotten to a place of balance with her thyroid as soon as in the past, with medication and also simply a few lifestyle changes, yet then life occurred. She and also her spouse expanded their company and also responsibilities ended up being requiring. She let what benefited her escape, her health was no more a priority in relation to various other much more pressing needs.

In the middle of all of it, her body was sending out up smoke signals and alarm bells were sounding. Her heart started to race once again, and her eye signs began to proceed. Still, she really did not do the important things that had actually worked in the past. So, that's why she called me. She needed a train, she needed someone to support her on, hold her liable, offer her love, and also remind her of her skills as well as strengths.

As you popular, it is so hard to undergo this alone.

It has taken me two years to get to business of creating this tool set down and devoting it to something more than my mercurial memory. I understand there will certainly be times in my life to come when I will certainly require to hear this pep talk once again, as well as I wish to hear it stated in a loving way.

I'm truly creating this book because I have actually been with a collection of life's difficulties over the last few years as well as the very same symptoms maintain showing up. Every single time I go through something that stresses me out, I feel my aspects of the illness expand and obtain stronger. I know precisely what it seems like to have a thyroid flare. I recognize, due to the fact that I have actually gone from being normal with the occasional flare, to being incredibly active with degrees 7 times with they should be, to being method hypothyroid, to after that ping-ponging up until getting here somewhere stabilized between.

It's a wonderful place to be in the middle. It's like you're on your own once again and you really feel strong and also excellent, and also certain and then situations alter. It remains in minutes when scenarios alter that I locate medicine to be tricking. It guarantees balance and also shelter, but it is really extra akin to a purgatory. It is unreliable since it is the only constant in an ever-changing circumstance. It doesn't respond to your body, your body replies to it. So, along with battling a disease, my body needed to battle the symptomatic actions to yet one more influence.

The day my medical professional sentenced me to a life on medicine, was the day I resolved to take procedures totally into my very own hands. I became my very own authority on my health and I made a plan 3 months later, I remained in remission.

Coping with Graves' Disease and Thyroid Eye Illness provided me a new vision, as well as a new method of locating equilibrium and focus in what had become a very dark and also complex world. Nothing looked real. The sides of points were fuzzy, as well as challenging to specify. I was lost.

Throughout this whole journey, when I have actually really felt less than strong, I have wanted someone to aid me see the future in a far better way. I have desired a pep talk as well as counsel when I forget my best self and also what brings me good health. I can not discover a true Tomb' Illness and Thyroid Eye Illness trainer, so I decided to become one. In becoming my very own train, I created a publication as well as I unlocked to assisting others.

My intention in writing this publication is to inspire as well as support recovery as well as lasting remission from Tomb' Disease and also Thyroid Eye Disease. It outlines what has helped me, as well as I am additionally going to share with you the tale of what helped Sparrow, as well. She is my client that achieved typical thyroid degrees within eight weeks of working with me as well as following my plan. I have a great suspicion that if you were to use these concepts, it might work for you, also.

Remission is absolutely as lovely and rejuvenating as it sounds. It resembles an oasis.

I wish this book inspires you to join me below, on this side of remission. If ever you require assistance or wish to reach out and also connect, simply email me at heathermaerussell@gmail.com. I will certainly react.

Chapter 2

Chapter 1: My Story.

Humbling Occasions Along the Way to Solving the Trouble.

It took me about 9 months to confess to myself that something was incorrect and also it had not been all in my head. It took me one more three months to detect myself as well as ask for the appropriate type of examinations. It took one more nine months to relocate via the health care protocol as well as reach a doctor that would prescribe the correct medication for a nursing mama. Things got pretty negative throughout that window of time.

I fought with a loss of muscle mass. I would certainly touch my arms and be able to get to right with to the bone. My muscles seemed like superficial sacks of sand. I had such poor trembles and muscle mass weak point that surviving twenty mins of yoga exercise was a genuine task.

Standard points that I had actually done a thousand times prior to came to be difficult. At one factor I can carry 2 gallons of water up two flights of staircases, no problem. But during that time I would get to the top of the stairs with my child in tow as well as wish to collapse. I would want to put down on the floor and also not rise, simply cry. Sweat pouring down my back, my heart racing, my legs trembling.

I remember this day really well. I did the stairs to our apartment and worried when I took my child off my body that I would not be able to hold her, my arms felt so weak. It was lunch time, and also I watched as the shakes in my hands were so extreme that I couldn't bring a little plastic spoon of avocado to her mouth. These tremors and sensations of weak point were like the final external proof of the shivering I had been experiencing on the inside for months as well as months, considering that prior to my baby was birthed.

I cleaned up, trying not to break as well as go down meals damp with soapy water. I put down with her for a snooze but could not sleep. My eye itched and ached, and these headaches were a daily thing I couldn't shake. I laid there and questioned what had actually occurred to transform me right into this unsteady, scared and stressed mess.

My eye was concrete and localized. It was easy to look up what may make it really feel the means it did. The results was among 2 things, an injury or a thyroid discrepancy. That began a course I adhered to of substantial study. I was on fire. My thoughts were lightening rapid and also I barely slept. It was the strangest blend of productive as well as afraid stress and anxiety. My research was so comprehensive it really felt scholastic. The drive recognized, evocative a few of the most difficult and satisfying periods in my life. Partially, this resemblancc is what made it so hard to see something was wrong, to put my finger on what was off to begin with.

Some people locate themselves first identified with some type of psychological inequality first. Bipolar, stress and anxiety, anxiety and so on are usually some of the first indications of thyroid inequality, yet individuals go initially to mental health physicians as well as at times it takes years for them to determine the resource of the imbalance as a thyroid issue. It is seriously that the mental as well as psychological side of Tomb' Illness and Thyroid Eye Illness is maybe the hardest component of everything. I have talked to females that spent time in psychiatric wards because their symptoms were mistakenly identified. Imagine how that must have felt!

Throughout the entire experience of these diseases, I have actually located anxiety as well as worry to be truth representatives of damage, as well as I assume these 2 things are what make some women seek aid in the first place. I'll be the initial to admit that when anxiety shows up, it turns up in the kind of a sign or a thyroid flare. It is like my physique calling for a break, a house call from my Greater Self. Frequently, it develops in the kind of my throat going tight. If I don't address the fearful idea soon enough, after that other physical signs and symptoms manifest. I have indicators I read.

My pinkie nail on my left hand will start to go white as well as peel far from the nail bed. For some reason, that is my inform. That is just how I know there is an underlying condition of illness that requires to be addressed. It shows up with other signs and symptoms, like anxiety or insomnia, or a twitchy eye.

At first, seeing these points once more entirely fanatics me out.

Initially it would over whelm me and afterwards I 'd just wait and also look for it to occur. I would certainly examine whether my remission was real, or if I had actually gotten on a deep state of imbalance. That question and also worry as well as worry would turn up, like the gas under the fire on a cooktop making whatever hot. I find that if I attend to the ideas and feelings when they show up, and go back to an area of nurturing and also forgiveness, after that the flare dissipates, the tension in my throat reduces as well as the headaches go away.

I can control the problem of my thyroid by regulating my feedback to the negative ideas that turn up. I can not avoid the thoughts from taking place, yet I can definitely release all previous point of view of the thoughts and also respond to them as though neutralizes their influence. In short, I can choose Large Love every which way. Training my mind to go where my heart leads is a method I pick everyday.

The everyday habits introduced right here are what assist me to utilize my mind as a tool of love. By using nutrients as well as acts of peace to this body which is the holy place for my heart, I use my spirit the ways to serve its objective: expressing Huge Love. It is so damn difficult to be caring and also light when you feel like the darkest components of heck. Stepping into love takes place one selection at a time. One act of Self Love at once.

I supply you encouragement on your trip, as well as support in times of requirement. There is clarity to be located on this path. Running hot and also seeing dual has actually gotten the job done of showing me that nothing is actual. That exactly how I see things is far more important that what I see. You might discover that if you close your eyes, have confidence, pick peace, produced the fire raging within you, that you, as well will locate cool relief in Large Self Love.

Chapter 3

Phase 2: The Big Option

Residence ablaze

Graves' Disease and Thyroid Eye Condition are autoimmune diseases. They are tough to identify and also increase with each other. I initially checked out autoimmune diseases resembling a wildfire in a post by Dana Trentini on October 30, 2014, titled, "Autoimmune Diseases Make in Your Body for YEARS Prior To Medical diagnosis." In her article, Trentini speaks about exactly how antibodies can build up in the body for several years before getting to a mentionable threshold in labwork. One autoimmune condition frequently brings about another (25% of those with one are most likely to develop others) as well as autoimmune problems grow early and also bloom like fires in a woodland filled with kindling. The magical variety of buildup is seven. Obtain diagnosed with one, and also seven is your potential future. Oh, and if you have children, keep a close eye on what happens when their hormonal agents begin to move, as this is when the initial indications of autoimmune antibodies appear.

That number is unacceptable to me. I understand that it is simply a number, which there is a feasible point of view that says, "Why separate? The feedback in all autoimmune illness is the same, we just distinguish based on the affected tissue."

I've had migraine headaches behind my appropriate eye since I was nineteen.

Migraines are an autoimmune condition (I had no idea until I began researching my thyroid). The year I turned nineteen was a tough year for me and the very first time I ever before went through what I involved take grown-up problems: My friend copulated my partner. I had a psycho roommate. I resided in a risky location with 4 men and also freaked my parents out totally. I barely passed courses in school. Every one of this gibberish abided with each other was a great deal to take care of for a former goodie-two-shoes, specifically while also living far from house for the first time and working as a semi-independent adult. It injured my head.

Part of what I realized when I started this trip to remission, was that I had already gotten three autoimmune diseases, starting with those very early migraine headaches. If I really did not disrupt whatever was going on, I 'd likely acquire even more. Like I stated, that was undesirable, as well as yet my research study was revealing boosting numbers of ladies over forty were pestered by autoimmune conditions.

I asked myself, "What can I do to stop the wildfire surging available?"

After that it hit me: the fire isn't available. It is shedding on the inside of my body! My body belongs to a home, as well as the fireplace of my house is a kitchen range. I cook each day. I can't not have the fire, I simply can not have it burning out of control.

This allegory of Tomb' Illness as a fire on the cooktop in your home is a clear aesthetic for me. Our thyroid regulates the body's temperature level. When our degrees are out of balance, we are commonly running warm, a little flighty and quicker tempered than we would certainly like with individuals. Being overheated is a classic sign and maintains us up in the evening. Our heart rates are much more than typical and we are anxious, anxious and also aggressive. We shiver and also relocate unpredictable methods.

When we are out of equilibrium, the fire has actually leapt off the stove and taken over our house.

Just how You Pick to Manage that Fire is Everything

Allow's truly push this metaphor of Tomb' Illness as a residence fire, one that is wearing out of control.

Imagine it's dinnertime as well as you are cooking. Your alone in the cooking area, yet the house is nuts with sound-- the pet, your kid's phone, your partner, the TV. You are making something good, perhaps fried chicken. The fire under the frying pan is as well warm, and also when it licks over the edge the poultry ignites.

Fizz, it obtains huge. Your house gets louder.

You just view it, interested at first, since it terrifies you a little. Because minute you have a couple of choices:

1. You not do anything, simply stand there changing your feet as well as wringing your hands, taking out your hair, eyes growing wide as well as incredulous. After that the house and also all you enjoy, the people and so on, go up in flames with you.

2. You turn on the fan expenses and watch, went crazy because somehow that makes the flames expand. You flick on the ceiling follower in

the dining room and open the sliding glass door. It's all you can consider. You start to swing a dishtowel over fires as well as smoke, however once more, that simply feeds the fire. After that the dishtowel ignites as well as stunned, you throw it. It captures the drapes ablaze. After that all of it occurs so rapid as well as house as well as all you like, individuals and more, rise in fires with you.

3. You utilize teacup of water after teacup of water, attempting to place the fire out. You tell your husband to collect the kids as well as leave. You just keep doing the same point over and also over, meager efforts to put out the raging fire in front of you, wishing it will certainly function, despite the fact that it is clear the fire is spreading out of control. After that your home goes up with you grasping the teacup in discouragement.

4. You get angry at your spouse for distracting you (he had actually simply shouted your name from the living room). It created you to transform your head and that's when the fire licked over the edge as well as established the frying pan ablaze. You can obtain so concentrated being upset with him as well as recounting the reasons why this occurs every single time, that you do not see when the flames catch the dishtowel on fire and that box of noodles. After that residence as well as all you love, the people and so forth, increase in flames with you, angry and suggest.

5. You phone call to your spouse and also claim, "Please provide me a minute." After that get the cover to the frying pan, put it on the fire, and also sink the whole point right into cold water. Then, you go join your other half in the living room and order take-out for everyone.

Here is the Solution

It is difficult to reach number 5.

I had to come to number five.

I had to discover a method to confine that fire as well as rejoin the crucial individuals in my life for something fun.

I spent three months creating significant shifts and achieving significant results.

I edited what was currently out there and functioning well for females with autoimmune conditions. I found a great deal of stuff on hypothyroid, but less on hyperthyroid. I filtered whatever through the special requirements I had. This was naturally filteringed system by what I recognized to be real at the time.

The outcome happened so fast it threw me off-guard, as well as I experienced a swing to the opposite hypothyroid side while I was still on medication. This is common even among clients who are just attempting to reach stablizing on drug. Accomplishing the right level is testing considered that the only constant in life is modification. I came to be extremely aware of what each side felt like, as well as maintained good track of feelings and feelings throughout those times too, so I had lots of information to note my progression with.

It took me 3 months to leave drug as well as I did it by utilizing these tools:

1. I followed Sarah Ballantyne's The Paleo Method, and also concentrated it on hyperthyroid demands, as well as abreast with my active life as a currently solitary working mama of a young daughter.

2. I committed to a day-to-day regimen of hygiene, massage, and timed cool showers.

3. I committed to an everyday yoga exercise splash as well as nature bath.

4. I created a daily technique of concentrated tranquility.

5. I successfully handle my physical, psychological, and also emotional symptoms with the fewest variety of specific supplements and successfully timed doses.

6. I keep excellent housekeeping behaviors within as well as a I have a strong Large Love practice.

I make use of these six things every day to keep the fire on the oven controlled as well as used for the best purposes. I do these points to make sure that I can change the flame of my thyroid I do the handles on my kitchen stove.

Since below is the thing: I'm in remission currently, and I have actually been for 3 years, however that does not mean it is long-term. In fact, I recognize it isn't a forever offer because I am so sensitive to what is taking place within, I can inform when there is also a tip of a thyroid flush. I recognize when that fire obtains the very least bit out of control as well as what circumstances I remain in when it occurs. That level of sensitivity is a survival device, comparable to a fire extinguisher, as well as it offers me the self-confidence I require to handle this disease successfully.

Dr. Kelly Turner utilizes the expression "extreme remission" and also has created a book by the same name. She recognizes 9 factors that contribute in creating these remissions:

1. Changing your diet plan
2. Organizing your health and wellness
3. Following your intuition
4. Using herbs and supplements
5. Releasing subdued feelings
6. Boosting positive emotions
7. Accepting social assistance
8. Strengthening your spiritual Connection
9. Having solid reasons to live

All of us read about near incredible healing or improvements in patients sentenced to a lifetime of drug-managed unhealthy state. The vital point is not to take any individual's word as an edict, rather view it as an opinion. Also if thyroid concerns run in one's family as well as also the disease has actually already shown up, epigenetics clarifies that also that which is created in genetics is not composed in rock. Genes expression (turning the genetics on and also off) can be manipulated and affected equally as the already materialized disease can be as well.

All of this indicate having a method to browse these expressions as well as discover to select the preferred expressions typically.

Sparrow

There have actually been hiccups along the road. As I strolled Sparrow via her initial 8 weeks, we obtained a good take a look at what challenges the procedure as well as impedes progression.

Actually, while most of the women I have interviewed have actually made a handful of dietary changes, those who dive into the autoimmune paleo diet plan with gusto as well as honest initiative have the biggest initial success with it. The majority of stick to dietary adjustments for about two months at the most, maybe 3, before they fall off of it as well as insinuate their consuming practices. I have actually slid on occasion, too. Specifically when my child and also I spent some time living with my moms and dads. I really did not intend to be the one that was so picky and also unusual, and so I curved my requirements and felt the influence almost right away.

On the various other hand, Sparrow really did not battle with the diet regimen in any way. Just when she took place vacation did it present an issue. While she gave in as well as ate a couple of fried clams with her family members in the method they do each year vacationing in this one area, she did it at a time when she was deeply unwinded, in a low stress and anxiety environment, as well as having a happy terrific time. The influence of slipping in her diet regimen was hardly recognizable.

On the various other hand, right before she took place vacation, there was a harder week. She had really felt excellent leading into week six as well as maintained to a rigorous diet regimen that week, but as life got thick, she diminished of the other components in her plan of self care as well as the result was a large serious step backwards.

Here is what we learned: food is the easy component. Decide to follow what is outlined the very easy method phase three as well as be finished with it. It is the self care routines that I created customized for her that give so much relief they can not be dismissed.

Ultimately, what we laid out with each other, and comply with day-to-day, is the most basic ways to an end.

Once more, I'm a single mama. Sparrow has three youngsters. Whatever your circumstance is, it is most likely that you require something that solves to the heart of the matter without taking in every last wave of your diminished attention period and power!

Whatever we do to take care of ourselves as well as go into remission demands to be reliable and efficient, but it does not need to look exactly like mine. The plan has aspects that for Sparrow happen in the early morning and for me take place in the evening, but right here is the thing: they happen.

Everyday. Because they cause enduring health as well as joy, as well as in the end have an impact equivalent to or above the food we eat.

Chapter 4

Chapter 3: Diet Plan-- Feeding the Fire or Starving It

Tomb' Illness Altered My Partnership with Food

For about eight years before I conceived I was a pretty rigorous vegan. Now and then I would certainly eat something that had actually been made with an egg, as well as I ate honey, yet beyond that, I was vegan. It functioned really well for me, as prior to maternity, I was what Ayurveda (conventional integrative Indian medicine) refers to as a Kapha body, made from planet and water, as well as being vegan assisted me incorporate a lot more fire and air into my diet plan to lighten me up and obtain me moving. If I were dispirited I would certainly consume a zesty meal as well as do a hot yoga exercise class to establish me straight.

I was the tough kind, more oak than willow tree, if you understand what I mean. I strove at maintaining any type of kind of graceful shape and never ever actually seasoned being "thin." When I ended up being vegan, it just functioned and truly made sense for my physique. I worked extremely well on that particular diet plan for several years.

As a matter of fact, I think a lot of women who plan pregnancies have a tendency to do so at once when they feel their finest or are in the very best shape of their lives. I was among those females. I didn't always intend it, but as quickly as I was open to the suggestion it occurred, and indeed, it was at a time in my life when I was more comfy in my own skin than I had actually been in a very long time.

Throughout my pregnancy I saw a midwife and also did not have a whole lot of blood work done. We did the minimum as there was no noticeable requirement for much more. I knew I was anemic, and also as a vegan that was not a surprise, so I supplemented with iron. I really felt extremely nervous, and also asked if that might be associated with anemia, yet from what I was reading regarding pregnancy and pregnant mommies, this was foregone conclusion anyhow. One of the most essential people in my life who had gone through maternity strengthened that messaging. So, I did what I have actually constantly done when it concerned really expressing what I was feeling, I attacked my tongue and also didn't state anything.

I raise all of this being vegan organization and anemia found during pregnancy since it resolves up a finer factor I failed to value at the time. I entered into that maternity currently in a problem of deficiency. The loss of blood throughout delivery intensified the issue. Recovering from all-natural childbirth and after that nursing were such big needs on my body that it totaled up to a great deal of compounded tension.

Throughout the first couple of months article partum, I went down a great deal of weight swiftly. I hadn't clued in yet, however my thyroid was truly revved during this moment. I was frequently starving as well as asked yourself if it was just the needs of nursing. The compliments on my gone down weight as well as how good I looked so soon after having a child, were totally up in arms with the method I really felt within. Foods that used to bring me hrs of energy as well as made me feel excellent were insufficient and also dismayed my food digestion.

Lengthy story short, I understood something wasn't right. Yet, I experienced the holiday season without addressing it: frequently hungry, eating empty calories due to the fact that they existed. If I got too hungry my head pain and also I would get incredibly discontented, so fudge was better than nothing.

My point with all of this is that I first new something was truly incorrect with me when my gut started going bad, however I waited to do anything about it till my eye bothered me. My digestion was off which was like an emergency alarm, yet I was too sidetracked to listen it.

That, and I was continuously dive bombing my system with tough artillery in the type of hidden gluten, beans, grains, spices that originate from seeds, nightshades, nuts, and soy.

Basically, every dish I ate was an act of battle on my body.

The even more research study I did about diet, as well as the a lot more I found out about autoimmune disease, the reasons, the things that aggravate the situation, and why, the more clear the picture I had of what was going on inside. The best source I found on the topic is Dr. Sarah Ballantyne's The Paleo Strategy, as well as her blog site, The Paleo Mom. She is such a specialist on the science of leaky intestine and also exactly how that must be attended to first when it involves living with autoimmune conditions.

I agree. Food is the something we have full control over. We knowingly pick which things to place in our mouths, as well as the way that digestion works, the whole chemistry of business starts with the initial preference. Good health begins keeping that front runner, and I was not making smart choices.

Make what you eat be about peace. Your intention is to give awesome alleviation to your whole body. You want to feel like you are unwinding your system from the inside out. The huge image is that we can understand what's taking place inside the body by reading signs and symptoms according to the components.

Hyperthyroidism is about air and fire and also it's likewise about things that feed that fire as well as fan the fires.

Think of the term inflammatory. The word fire is inside the word inflammatory. Autoimmune illness are about a swollen inner action to problem. It is an over reaction to inner conflict. Tomb' Disease is extremely explicit regarding this. It doesn't hide. It has to do with speed as well as heat and protective aggression, uncontrollable impatience.

Our remedy after that is mosting likely to be based in bringing that rate down to something workable, bringing that heat to a tolerable temperature as well as bringing hostility and impatience to a place of healthy and balanced excitement. What is usually challenging regarding medicine is that it is difficult to achieve a sustainable level for lasting remedy without extensive negative effects. For instance I was on PTU for a complete year as well as at the end of that year I was depressed, overweight, still nervous, unbelievably awkward, and also absolutely a stranger to myself. I have actually learned through trial and error that synthetic medication simulates a feeling of balance for as lengthy as problems stay the same. Yet, change is the only constant, as well as unfortunately, medicine just isn't smart sufficient to alter with us. For this reason, medication functions truly well as a symptomatic appeaser, good for as long as the problems inside as well as on the surface stay the exact same. In other words, it is basically a temporary solution.

It is necessary when regulating diet plan and also creating adjustment that you frequently ask for your degrees to be analyzed. I believe every six weeks it is a great idea to have your numbers run. At this moment, I don't care so much about numbers any longer, however in the starting it was nice to see those numbers entered a location of balance. After a while, the goal is to end up being delicate sufficient not to need to see it in black-and-white theoretically to understand where your levels are. You will reach a point where you will be listened and you'll comprehend when your body is over reacting to an internal conflict.

Furthermore, you will have the tools to call that overreaction down.

The Essentials

Why is diet so crucial? It is so important because it is that first act. It's the moment that you reach make a definitive choice. You get to make a best activity in line with your health and wellness. While our immune system is a complex symphony of intelligent, innate as well as adoptive reactions involving our entire body, in streamlined way we can state that concerning 70 percent of it lives in our intestine. Diet regimen then becomes a great place to begin creating balance in our bodies. Sarah Ballantyne's book, The Paleo Technique is outstanding. It is my primary resource when it concerns diet plan, however it is thick as well as I located it a sincere challenge to read when my vision was at its worst.

There is so much significant scientific research behind the reality that leaky intestine is a major factor to autoimmune illness. Particularly several of the representatives that create leaking gut, are additionally specifically aggravating for Tomb' Condition patients. (If you connect to me at heathermaerussell@gmail.com, I'll take a look at the shape of your lips and also we will certainly know if you have a leaky intestine.) The factor for this is when you have the condition of dripping digestive tract, which autoimmune condition individuals on average do, tiny fragments of food primarily get away with your intestinal tracts and go into the rest of your body. They are taken into consideration international, so your body assaults these agents. The ironic point is, points like gluten actually look a lot like your thyroid hormonal agents so when you have particulates of gluten essentially just free roaming your body, it resembles a chemical bombing and your body goes on like hyper protection and also your immune system starts assaulting all of these foreign agents.

So you can choose because minute when you're about to take a bite of that donut, to knowingly prevent an act of war. The food you put into your body launches a chemical reaction which chain reaction is either one of healing and also love or basically protective strike as well as worry. Choose to only consume food that's mosting likely to help your body repair and reconstruct.

I suggest acquiring a duplicate of Sarah Balantyne's book The Paleo Technique as well as concentrating on phase 2 and all of the pages that use run-throughs of nutritional suggestions and also why. I am also a member of a number of Facebook Teams that share AIP dishes. Right here are the fundamentals of what to prevent as a person whose body immune system is assaulting the thyroid and eyes:

1. Grains.

2. Gluten.

3.Pseudo-grains and also grain-like materials.

4. Dairy.

5. Legumes.

6. Refined veggie oils.

7. Processed food chemicals as well as components.

8. Added sugars (consists of honey and also syrup in addition to pseudo-sugars).

9. Sugar alcohols.

10. Nonnutritive sweeteners (consists of stevia).

11. Nuts as well as nut oils (coconut is an exception).

12. Seeds and seed oils.

13. Nightshades or flavors derives from nightshades.

14. Spices that come from seeds.

15. Eggs.

16. Alcohol.

17. Coffee.

18.High-glycemic lots foods.

Wow. Doesn't that checklist look like it erases the modern diet plan as we have familiarized it? Well, that's since it does, and that's why it's call Paleo. What is the take home message right here? Reduce, simplify. Adhere to meats and also veggies, skilled with great oils, natural herbs, and also pink salt.

Sadly, I'm not specifically innovative when it pertains to recipes and also food preparation. That becomes part of the reason I had to generate a sustainable system for food on this diet plan. I am a solitary mama and also I have a young little girl. Cooking is something that I do at the end of the day when I am exhausted as well as starving.

So whatever I am making has to be simple, and ideally a one pot meal or a one pan dish. It's reached be something that I can assemble swiftly ahead of time if I need to, and also store in the fridge for an hour or more. I'm not client when it concerns dishes with multiple steps that need to be well timed. I use a lot of herbs because they are simple, cooling and they give great taste without originating from a seed.

I such as coconut oil to prepare with, olive oil to clothe with, as well as lemon. I have come to see points like wonderful potatoes and also mushrooms and other sweet vegetables like summer season squashes or wintertime squashes as well as stuff like that as artificial sweetener so I can keep my glycemic degrees low.

It has actually simply opened me approximately the easy enjoyment of sampling entire foods once again. There are a few points I continually struggle with, like coffee. I love coffee. However Sarah Ballantyne recommends that you maintain it to a cup of normal coffee daily. Since is simply a covering suggestion for autoimmune problems in general. Allow's bear in mind that Graves' Condition means we are currently over energetic people. For the first three-month duration where you're actually planning to developing a condition of repair rather than attack, it's important to do as lots of points as you can starting today to regulate, amazing as well as calm your system. Points like raised heart price, shivers, anxiety, tense nerves-- every one of those points are aggravated by the rate of caffeine. So I needed to taper down gradually to a location where I really did not have coffee routinely. Then I maintained that for 3 months. As soon as I accomplished a problem of balance, I reestablished it in little amounts on occasion. I appreciate it a lot, it is a true treat, and also it is well worth awaiting.

The Difficulty of Social Consuming.

Allow's talk about the treats, the Unpleasant No-nos for a minute or more. I state that term with caring fondness, as it was coined by among my dear friends from graduate college. It is what she described breads as: Unpleasant No-Nos.

We would certainly satisfy for coffee and NNs as well as relax.

It was our method to destress and I linked almond croissants with this notion for several years. The issue with that said is Unpleasant No-Nos are ruled by gluten.

All grains generally are to be avoided as a result of the manner in which they're refined (typically with glutenous things) and also since they create openings in the lining of your intestines. This sounds rude, but if you consider your poop and also can see the grains you ate the day in the past as almost entire units, after that you have essentially simply run a cord brush via your intestinal tracts and create a lot of mini splits.

Spices that come from seeds often tend to generate warmth in the body, and so do nightshades. Ayurveda recommends Pitta bodies, or fire bodies prevent nightshades and also fire causing flavors or astringent tastes, things that are mosting likely to produce a great deal of warm in your body or a great deal of air. This makes sense, since we intend to develop a feeling that is awesome and also refreshing within, not inflamed and gusty.

One that is deep and also tranquil, and that will certainly put earth on that fire you have actually got burning on your kitchen area range your in house. In home economics I was shown to place sodium bicarbonate on a fire and also placed the lid on the pan. What we want to do place sand on that fire and also blow out the fires. We desire amazing, refreshing, and earthy components.

Every one of this was so counterproductive to me before being pregnant. I was the exact opposite. I prevented points that were cool as well as rejuvenating as well as earthy since they made me dispirited. There was a home window of time after I had my child where I was actually feeding the flames. I was doing what had worked previously. I was producing a great deal of air in system with food and anxiety, as well as I was creating a great deal of heat. I was quick-tempered and angry. I really felt horrible as well as I didn't recognize what was going on within. I handled it in the most effective way that I knew exactly how.

The trouble was, I fell short to review the indications, and also truly take note. I chalked a great deal of it up to simply being a brand-new mom as well as never ever having actually done this previously. I wish I would've spoken out. I want I would've informed somebody about just how I really felt on the within.

I'm so delighted that I responded the way I finished with my endocrinologist appointed me that life sentence. It was the first time I bank on myself when it came to these illness. Sarah Ballantyne's publication was the initial publication I check out and knew would certainly benefit me. Executing it was an entirely various tale. She advises that you eat a variety of different foods consisting of cuts of meat and also the means you prepare them. I was so crazy with her suggestions as well as had the very best of purposes when I started.

But, I had a trouble, a challenge. I was ill as well as I did not have energy and also I lacked creativity. I'm not a foodie to begin with, and also I have a tendency to pick dishes that take less than half an hour to both prepare and cook. I'm willing to move a bit on the last however I need to have the ability to damage it up into stages. I have so many other points I would rather choose to do then chef. I do not also like to grocery store. Yet, I absolutely enjoy it when other individuals prepare for me.

That is part of the reason I fell off of this diet regimen. I met a person I was so ecstatic about-- I'm still truly delighted about him-- as well as he loves to cook for me. The trouble is he enjoys utilizing things that I can not eat. I tried. I spent the first year getting to know him as well as breaking my diet plan. I ate as best as I might when I was by myself or with my little girl, however when I went out with him as well as we ate in restaurants, or he prepared for me, I really did not intend to be "that lady." I really did not wish to be the one who claims, "I can't consume anything on the menu below tonight. Nope I'm not also going to have one taste of what you ordered for supper. I'm actually happy with this poached poultry and steamed veggies.".

Rather, I relaxed and I enjoyed myself and got to know he or she. At the same time, I additionally relocated right into my own house with my little girl, as well as wound up going through the following revolution of life's difficulties. Throughout the whole procedure my equilibrium within this disease and also my connection with it has actually been challenged.

I acknowledge that I'm never ever really mosting likely to be able to come off of this diet regimen. I additionally recognize that the extra I stick to it, the a lot more creative I end up being regarding appreciating it and also establishing brand-new favorite foods. I can additionally see the larger picture when it comes to seeing food as medication. The stomach is located right around the same location as your third chakra which is your power chakra. The high quality of food we eat is akin to eating the energy of the sunlight.

The power of the universe is within me and the whole foods that I eat can be carried into self-confidence, self-confidence, and the nerve to fulfill life's on a daily basis difficulties.

Our connection to power goes to the core of our health and wellness. If we ingest vulnerable processed food, we rob our bodies and compromise them.

Daily Diet Regimen Routine.

So what do I do? What is my daily diet regimen like? How do I follow the requirements of The Paleo Technique as well as still browse all the responsibilities of my life? This is an excellent concern. It is among the hardest things I do on a daily basis, and I can inform you that when I don't turn up daily, life starts to obtain hard. If I make thoughtless selections, they have consequences.

So I am the very first to admit that generally, I am extremely boring when it pertains to my diet.

I have 3 various dishes that I make use of for breakfast meatballs. I revolve them. It's enough variety for me if I also include leftovers for breakfast. Especially when I think about family members dishes. I have a tendency to consume morning meal by myself, regarding forty-five mins after I awaken (much more on my everyday modus operandi in the next phase). So this is very easy. When I eat morning meal with my little lady, or in a group of people, I prepare or bring the things I would like to consume.

Sarah Ballantyne advises two or three big dishes a day. No snacking. The reason for this is to support blood sugar level, and enhance food digestion. You want to give your body time to absorb a total dish prior to bringing new food into the formula. It has to do with secretions and also chemistry.

Food undergoes a cycle during food digestion and if you are adding something fresh to a cycle that has practically completed, some part of the procedure will certainly be interrupted, as well as intestine problems materialize.

I normally consume at least one salad a day. I make certain that there are always dark leafy eco-friendlies, either kale or spinach or arugula or something richer to contribute to Romain. I utilize Romain lettuce due to the fact that it has a nice crisis and also it's rejuvenating. I almost always grate a carrot and a quarter of a raw beetroot. That's where I get some of my sugar throughout the day. Then I have cucumbers, due to the fact that they are refreshing as well as cooling. Very same point for clothing: just olive oil, a little lemon juice, pink salt. I additionally utilize fresh herbs, often parsley in some cases cilantro. Anything that will certainly give the salad flavor like a dressing would certainly. Then I include poultry, fish or any type of type of meat. It's not always exciting, yet it's trusted, and also it's also something you can make in advance and take with you any place you're going.

Supper is the dish that I formally cook for my household. So today it's simply me and also my little lady, but sometimes we have a guest. Now the majority of my pals know that I have a restricted diet regimen, which I'm going to prepare the same point for every person. So they likewise understand that when they come to eat at my home they're going to leave sensation great as well as without regret the following day.

Supper is generally baked, steamed or sautéd. I don't have time for a lot more unless I intend thoroughly. Once a week, I like to prepare a whole poultry in the oven. It creates a good dinner with guests, or my little girl as well as I share it and then there's poultry for salad the next day. If I have much less time after that I just cook chicken legs or chicken upper legs or often fish or pork tenderloin. As you recognize I make a great deal of meatballs for morning meal so in some cases we have those for dinner on the day that I make them. This is typically where I start to incorporate beef. Beef is a heavy meat for me so I actually attempt to consume it each time when I have a good waking window to absorb it well. Normally that goes to breakfast.

My suggestion on adhering to the AIP Paleo diet is to streamline it as much as feasible. It doesn't imply that you need to sacrifice flavor, if you keep selection high there should not be an issue. For those people that aren't imaginative in the kitchen area, live alone, or couldn't care less about cooking, the less complicated, easier, as well as faster the better. It's a little bit of adjustment in the starting just get to a place where are you are no longer grabbing something packaged or quick to make that is refined. When you're over that obstacle every little thing else is easy.

So let me be clear here, even if a refined thing is organic, it's actually no great. Our objective right here is to restore our system. To boost our inner gastrointestinal power. So the reason plants and also whole foods are so essential, is since they are crucial. They have vigor, power from the sun made show. They are living breathing entities, who after that move the living breathing energy they have saved into you when you consume them. If something experiences a conditioning, or a processing, of any type of kind, after that you're currently lowering the vitality of that food. Now you require every little bit of power you can absorb while you restore the walls of your intestinal tracts, which have actually been permeated by intensifying entities, and after that remain to keep their good condition.

Try not to worry a currently stressed out system. There is no need to absorb something that isn't going to simply make it sing. Eat well as well as the information from natural veggies as well as top quality meats, fish, and fowl will certainly strengthen you. Choose a range of different cuts, to make sure that the distinct details stored in those areas nourishes you.

Opportunities are if you have ever before taken a yoga class your educator has pointed out the ways in which we save experiences as well as info in our joints, tendons and our muscular tissues around my body. The same holds true for pets. So select the information from pets that have an impressive experience in life. Your health depends on buying top notch products, so that no time at all is thrown away, to make sure that your body has exactly what it needs in order to re-create excellence.

Now that being stated, we're not speaking about a large quantity of food here, so while it is at first pricey to make this change, I have actually discovered that it evens out. I locate that the big meal described in Sarah Ballantyne's publication, is not that large. She's rather clear on that. Taxing your digestive system past its comfort level, is not contributing to its health.

Since our group tends to run quick, I located it was much better to really ground myself with 3 moderate dishes, and I avoid snacking entirely when possible.

Morning meal has actually constantly been my biggest difficulty. Making breakfast something that occurs within the initial half hr or so of being awake was an obstacle at first. After that I developed a great morning routine that lands me at breakfast within about forty-five mins of waking up.

Food doesn't have to be dressed up as well as gently refined to be appealing. It just is appealing. Entire foods are attractive. Animals are intelligent and stylish, as well as plants are remarkable as well as solid. As a former vegan I truly needed to cover my heart around approving the present that animals bring to the table. The work that they have actually done to turn their flesh as well as bone into nutrient abundant material loaded with honesty and planetary power is extraordinary. I needed to reach a location where I can accept that grant a clear conscience as well as light heart. Considering it by doing this made it possible for me to go from not having had meat for over eight years, since I was vegan for a few years prior to ending up being vegan, to consuming meat 3 times a day.

When I was still on drug and also headed toward remission I was truly strict concerning my diet. I utilized to bring my very own Himalayan pink salt with me anywhere I went. Yes, I was that girl! Below's things: being that lady helps me. When I make sure I take good treatment of myself I feel extra like myself.

If I obtain laid-back about it as well as have some chips and salsa one evening (due to the fact that I'm depriving and also I'm out to supper with my partner) I'm dive- bombing my system. Nightshades, seasonings, and also grains are an essential mix of things that create an extreme issue. Perhaps I also give in as well as have a margarita. The next early morning I can inform promptly that I have actually just infected my body. I can see it in the swelling around my eyes. I can see it in the swelling around my ankles. And also I can feel it in my state of mind. I'm pissed, warm, distressed. I'm restless. I'm tough on myself since I've simply barged in my diet plan. I'm chewing at the little bit, waiting to snap.

I am a house ablaze.

Yet, suppose you wish to have a social life, like to travel, or if you are single and you want to date? Heck, what if you simply desire a night off?

What do you do when you're eating out? At first, I struggled to be social because my diet plan was restricted as well as "no enjoyable." That resulted in a descending spiral in self-confidence and isolationism (we will certainly talk A LOT a lot more concerning that later). For now, let's just speak about the fact that it is nearly impossible to head out to consume! So, here's what I do: I request for a salad without tomatoes or dressing and afterwards request for olive oil and also lemon on the side. I keep it simple, maybe ask to add barbequed hen, no oil. Dining establishments often tend to use cheap oils we need to prevent, so be clear concerning this when ordering.

It can be very easy if you locate complete satisfaction in simpleness as well as knowing that you are making a good selection. The result of which will last longer than the short-term preference of something poisonous.

Every single time I placed something in my mouth I am selecting to experience war or peace. Basically, it comes down to that. Feed the fire or starve it. When you remain in a state of inequality, think about it this way. There is no alternative. Food is the truest medication.

Below is my guidance: Go with what works. Learn the things to stay clear of, and also make sensible choices. Simple is as good as a banquet: keep to this policy and also you'll do well and also stay with the procedure.

Right here's another piece of diet plan recommendations: go done in. Sarah Ballantyne says the same thing. Go done in for three months and also stay with it. You will certainly create a distinction.

One note on supplements: I take a multivitamin for ladies over forty, 200mg of Selenium (helpful for eyes), and a teaspoon in water of diatomaceous earth day-to-day (great for hair as well as nails).

Now, allow's take a look at just how to further nourish ourselves as we undergo adjustment as well as restoration.

Chapter 5
Chapter 4: Creating Healthy Patterns

G.R.A.V.E.S

. A lot of important individuals have morning rituals that are at the heart of their success. I took that easy concept and kept up it. I required a means to obtain my butt out of bed. Apologies for the blasphemy, yet that is as basic as it gets. In the very first 3 months of establishing these practices, I was so out of equilibrium as well as depressed that by the time I would ultimately dropped off to sleep in the very early hrs of the morning, I would only remain asleep for about three or four hrs before my daughter awakened and the day started. I wanted to weep before I had actually even seen the light of day.

Part of what I learned about caring for myself when I was identified, is that the method I begin the day affects the remainder of the day ahead. Launching a problem of remainder in which repair work can happen begins first thing.

Deepak Chopra states in Quantum Recovery that if one wants to bring back the body's very own recovery capacity, whatever needs to be done to bring it back into equilibrium. Deep leisure is one of the most vital precondition for treating any disorder. The goal is to come to a regular condition of remainder.

Okay, allow's be frank, when I initially checked out these words, I thought. "Fat chance. I remain in a constant state of panic and also impatience is my way of life." Accomplishing a regular problem of remainder is way simpler stated than done.

Specifically if your body is surging as well as going seven times faster than it normally would.

It made excellent feeling, however, and I knew if I took the actions I needed to, in order to reduce, I would certainly at the very least obtain near a condition of remainder.

This was more than a physical modification for me. It indicated a review of my worths and beliefs. Rest was a bad word in my book. It indicated negligence and an absence of productivity. Like I stated, I was a heater.

I utilized to delve into my day with a massive mug of coffee. I would certainly attempt to obtain as much work performed in the morning as possible, and then be tired by mid mid-day. I would certainly have an additional large cup of coffee and after that continue working up until previous dinner time. After that, when I had my little woman, and my thyroid really revved, I would certainly awaken so worried, so frustrated, and also stressed concerning whatever it would certainly paralyze me. I was remarkably sidetracked (a lot so I really felt insane) and incapable of resting still. My body shivered as well as my limbs shivered, ready to fight or run at any kind of moment.

Afterwards eventful meeting with my endocrinologist, and also I got serious about looking after myself, I recommended a slow motion morning ritual. While it is a difficulty to sustain it, specifically with a little kid, it is worth every min I awaken earlier than she does. It is sacred time, as well as sanity time.

Like a lot of early morning routines, I've mapped this one according to an phrase:

G: rise, get still, get quiet R: reflect

A: attest V: envision E: exercise S: silence

G: Rise. That's right. Just turn one leg at a time over the edge as well as obtain your body out of bed willingly. Often this is so damn hard! However do it, as well as do it with thankfulness. Fake it up until you make that gratitude actual. Every day my alarm system goes off at 4:20 in the morning It's really part of the bedtime application on my phone. So instead of an actual alarm I awaken to the audio of birds chirping. This has entirely emotionally altered the method I think about waking up to an alarm. I do not make myself wake up on the crack of a whip, yet it feels better to stand up within a couple of minutes of the alarm system going off. Now, if it takes much longer, as well as it feels like a hard morning, that is okay, because I've budgeted sufficient time for myself. Now you could be thinking that voluntarily getting out of bed at 4:20 in the early morning is simply bat crap insane. I listen to that however below's the important things: it's not. It's a little tough to get used to it first, but once you do, that sacred time in the early morning is something you anticipate. You have actually sculpted it out just for you. (Later on I discuss shutting off alerts on your phone from 8pm to 8am, so this time around in the early morning is genuinely continuous.).

I get up and head straight for the shower room. The first thing I do is oil pull. I keep sesame oil in a pump bottle by the hand soap and squirt a few times into my mouth. This seems so gross, best? You'll get utilized to it, and also can mix in a rejuvenating necessary oil if it assists you do this. The advantages of oil pulling are numerous so do a quick net search regarding it's detoxing abilities. Roll the oil around in your mouth for regarding ten minutes while you feed the cat as well as put some hot water on boil. Then spit the oil out into the toilet and scrape your tongue. I use a stainless-steel tongue scrape as well as I do it before I have actually even had a sip of water or comb my teeth. In the evening your gastrointestinal system cleans and toxins build up on the surface of your tongue. If in the early morning you are searching in the mirror and also you stick your tongue out, and also it's covered with a white film, then that's a sure sign that you're eating something that doesn't agree well with you. It's a terrific means to judge food allergies and intolerances as well as inequality in general. After I have actually scuffed my tongue, I clean my teeth as well as use a little sesame oil to massage therapy my eyes. I carefully scrub the oil across my eyelids and around the orbits. I locate this really aids with fuzzy vision that comes from completely dry eyes.

After that I head to the kitchen, drink a huge glass of space temperature filtered water, and make tea. The tea I drink in the early morning is turmeric based. I take a heaping half a tsp of turmeric and a great dash of cinnamon as well as pour boiling water over them. In the initial three months of following the AIP diet, it is suggested that you do not make use of any kind of sugarcoated. I couldn't consume this tea at first, so I started by including a little taste of honey and also utilizing less as well as much less everyday. Now I consume it without anything and also actually like the taste.

While the tea is soaking, I consume alcohol around 4 ounces of aloe vera juice. I swish it around my mouth, under my tongue as well as around my periodontals. I swish it and also ingest. Once again, a quick internet search will light up the dental health and wellness benefits of aloe, and also the anti-inflammatory benefits of turmeric extract. Then I grab my tea and I head for my reflection padding. I roll out my yoga floor covering as well as take a seat. I light a candle light and also beverage slowly. I being in silence for a couple of mins, simply getting into the groove. I have one objective during this time. All I do is observe the thoughts that cross my mind, and placed a gold star next to the ones that are positive. I line up with the gold stars.

Just how would certainly I deal with this if I really did not have a yoga floor covering, or meditation padding or actually if I hadn't ever before even given either of those a shot? Well, I would sit in a nice chair with a cup of tea and also view the dawn. Among my clients chosen remaining on the sofa first thing in the early morning with a reflection playing. The point is, she stands up, gets still, as well as she obtains silent. These things come first.

R: Reflect on all the important things that are going right. Those shiny gold stars alongside every one of the effective ideas need to build up. If it is difficult to see that, after that take the following five thoughts and compose them down in 3 words or much less. I maintain a stack of sticky notes and also 3 x 5 index cards alongside my reflection station as well as use them as necessary. I put my notes right into one of two piles: those I give a gold star, as well as those I do not.

If my mind starts right away competing, then I'll call a reflection on my phone. But also for me this is the last option.

Opening my phone is like opening Pandora's box. It's something I avoid up until the last moment feasible. I have set my phone to do not disturb from 8 PM to 8 AM. I don't obtain any work notifications or things like that between those hours. Sparrow is a dining establishment owner as well as when I first asked her to establish her alerts to these times, she really did not think it was feasible. But upon reflection she acknowledged that she felt like she never left job. She felt like she never ever had a break. Points might not take place without her responses. I asked her to just try it, to just tell her people that that's what she was mosting likely to do as well as do it. It functioned. So currently when she gets up in the early morning, she has virtually 3 hours before somebody else is mosting likely to ask her to do something.

This morning ritual has to do with waking up and doing something for yourself first. Self-care initially. Then caring for others is very easy.

This quiet time of reflection is when we start to see patterns in our lives. Creating a gratefulness list appears so obvious that I'm often temped to neglect it, however it's additionally one of one of the most effective devices I have for seeing the positive side. If I'm having an early morning where the negative cards are extra plentiful than the positive cards, after that I write out at the very least 3 brand-new things I'm grateful for. I have my attempted as well as trues, my go-tos, individuals I like and so on, yet with this workout I get refined. I consider the little things that make my day wonderful, and I create them down in a different way every day. I feel the gratitude in my heart and then let it go. I write down things like, "I am so grateful for the gift of this unique view. I am so grateful for this uncommon point of view and the wisdom it brings. I am so grateful to see my life via the eyes of love and also not fear. I am so thankful that to recover is to content. I am so happy I can do anything I placed my heart and mind to." I do this quickly, due to the fact that if I do not, wonderful ends up being depressing in a fraction of a second. So relocating through that gratitude as well as launching the darkness side of it is a choice I make before it also comes up.

A: Affirmation. The appreciation list is my means of starting a pep talk to myself. I discover the methods which I are in charge of bringing that which I'm so thankful for right into being. Self affirmation doesn't come naturally to me, so I grow my listing with some good analysis. A few of my favored books today:.

Quantum Recovery by Deepak Chopra, Anatomy of the Spirit by Carolyn Myss, A Training Course in Miracles, A Training Course in Miracles Made Easy by Alan Cohen, as well as Go Back To Love by Marianne Williamson.

I normally invest regarding 20 mins reading. Certainly a couple of lines always attract my focus and they will certainly influence my favorable affirmation for the day. I compose this down. There is something extremely connectively powerful concerning placing your intention and your affirmation down in your very own handwriting. Seeing in your script words that affirm the direction you wish to enter is no little matter. Make them your own and possess the power inherent in them. I'm a crier, and also locate that when I am at my most at risk vigorously, basic words have an extensive affect. Launching stress via tears is a relief as well as while it was really hard at first to be so absurd, I now find wonderful enjoyment in launching that lump in my throat that originates from intending to cry over something or everything. (More on this later on.).

Via affirmations that prove out, we come to have a clearer idea of what it is we value and think. If something makes us intend to cry due to the fact that we either desire that so much for ourselves, or due to the fact that we were when because state, or we don't assume it is feasible again, then that is something to bear in mind of. Create it down in black and white so you can provide yourself that very same affirmation again and again throughout your day. I have a tendency to use a lot of Post-It notes or 3x5 index cards, and Sharpies. I such as to see them in popular locations any place I go. On the shower room mirror, on the front door, above the range in the kitchen area, peppered across my job desk.

Right here are a few of the affirmations I have actually got up today: "Make your mind an instrument of love.".

" Step out of self consciousness and right into self acceptance." "Hey, gorgeous, you have actually got great eyes as well as see wonders all over.".

V: Visualization. Take a couple of mins to put those positive affirmations right into purpose setting. Write these things down, as well as what typically happens is they will certainly launch a visualization. For instance the affirmation, "Make your mind a tool of love," morphed into, "I untangle impulses of fear, and also weave love rather." After that I invested the following stretch of time envisioning myself resting at a loom. I tint coded the worry as warm and also mad and also red, and chose that this tapestry I'm weaving was indicated to be of awesome blues, eco-friendlies, silvers, as well as soft golds. So I imagined myself taking out the red fearful threads and also changing them with trendy blue strings, and nurturing environment-friendly strings. After that I stood back from the tapestry and also saw a tale woven in, it was my life, loaded with calm purposeful activity.

Actually, what I could not see when I looked exterior, I can see with terrific clarity when I looked inward.

E: Exercise. These favorable affirmations as well as visualizations commonly result in powerful sensations. The best way that I understand to actualize and externalize that powerful sensation, is a twenty minute yoga exercise blast (prevent compressing the front of the neck). This blast makes reveal the effective objectives I have envisioned. I exercise my greatest capacity in deliberate, conscious action. If this happens in the form of a walk or series of stretches you like or a self massage therapy (see below), it doesn't matter. What matters is that you release that effective sensation into the world, understanding that energy begets power as well as you are going to recover and also nourish your body with effective food, ideas, and also actions throughout the day.

I don't consider this exercise in the typical feeling of the word. It isn't jogging, it isn't cardio calorie burning or a targeted elimination of fat.

There are a variety of courses to select from and designs of yoga to check out. Choose one valued on a spiritual level, not just a physical degree.

I've done a lot of various styles of yoga exercise over the last twenty years, and also checked out a large range of choices. Before my little girl was birthed, I chose yoga exercise in a cozy area. It helped me exercise my twists and get looser much faster. After she was born, as well as I began to feel off, I returned to what had actually helped me before. I did brief extreme methods while she snoozed as well as tried to give myself power by feeding that fire within, believing that my depression was an outcome of torpidity and the weight I had actually obtained during pregnancy. But all that did was take the fire that was stressing out of control on the inside and follower the flames. I was a sweating trembling mess by the end of a twenty minute method. It was a dramatic contrast to the stamina and power I had actually previously really felt as a result of what had worked well for me prior to.

Via experimentation, expedition of several different online sources, and learning more about what my body needed to cool down and also get solid once again, I picked staying clear of any type of warm yoga, and also dedicated to twenty minutes a day of very slow-moving flow combined with corrective aspects. Today, I just wake up as well as relocate a manner in which feels good, that brings type to the power I feel within when I write my affirmations down and also imagine realising them.

I exercise my power, and therefore, extend and also strengthen that power within. Yoga is such an efficient device for this, because at the same time, you are breathing deeply, relocating your body in symbolic ways, as well as squeezing as well as pressing body organs so they can launch as well as regulate.

In the initial stages of changing my diet regimen, I thought of all of these floating particulates of gluten and also little bits of food drifting around in my system, leaking out of my digestive tracts. Yoga exercise eliminated what I viewed as particles, much like the particles in a home jumbled with dirty nicknacks and also flammable ornaments. I find that the very same point can happen if I do a twenty minute walk outside or stand barefoot in the yard for awhile.

S: Silence. At the end of my method, I hum for a very long time. I just take a deep breath as well as hum, reduced in my throat and also calm my thyroid with noise therapy. After that I sit in silence and allow all that has come previously in the morning settle into my heart. I find it is simplest to practice meditation in earnest at this time. The restlessness I feel first thing in the early morning sweetens and also I can concentrate breathing with my thyroid with clarity and also objective.

Chapter 6.

Chapter 5: Clearing Up the Debris You Can See.

Detoxing the Body.

Purging the toxins accumulated in the body though yoga exercise, or mild exercise of power, is a whole lot like spring cleaning your home. Changing my diet helped me to make certain that I would not collect even more particles, but I needed multiples means to remove what had currently gathered.

I approached this issue from the angle of asking what are one of the most efficient methods to put out a fire? Whenever I go camping, I generally extinguish a fire by putting water on it. Consuming a gallon of water a day assists me to clear toxic substances from my body that are water soluble. It hydrates my skin, and when my thyroid was burning the midnight oil, it seemed like my skin was dry and wrinkling faster than ever. Remaining moisturized not just gives my skin a supple quality from the inside out, it additionally helps me to have better energy, psychological professors, and excellent state of mind policy.

After flooding the flames with water, I typically shovel sand into the fire pit to stifle the coals. It is the final action I constantly take to be sure that the coals are chilly and absolutely nothing can mistakenly smolder and burst into flames later. There is constantly that final burst of heavy steam that the dying fire lets off prior to it goes silent. It is different that the heavy steam that comes when you put water over it. I think the same is true wherefore occurs to that inner inferno when you drink water, consume well, and after that additionally find a method to pull particles out via your skin.

Doesn't that noise so gross, yet good?

The skin is our biggest body organ. If you consider the gastrointestinal system as one huge lengthy tube with openings at each end, then transform that whole tube right into a donut as well as see your skin as the exterior. It is a torus shape, similar to the waves for power that emit outside from heart facility. Diet nurtures the donut's opening, and also oil massage therapy nurtures the rest.

In the evening, prior to I go to bed, I do an Ayurvedic massage using coconut or sesame oil. In the summertime I utilize coconut because it isn't as warming, and because it reminds me of sunscreen! The whole process I'm going to describe below audios rich, and it is. It has to do with the healing power of touch as well as providing your skin, the largest body organ in your body, enrichment and also a means for it to draw toxins out of within. I have a towel I've marked for this objective, as well as daily I spread it out on the restroom flooring. I scoop a fifty percent a tablespoon right into my hand as well as let the oil melt as I spread it throughout my skin.

I begin with my face and scalp. Utilizing my fingertips, I bring blood as well as feeling to the top of my head. I roll in circle my eyes and also across my cheekbones as well as jaw. I use a certain rhythm, order and also course for this. I move in circles as well as figure forms. I treat my eyes with love and care. I advise myself of what a gift it is to see, to see within, to understand that this special sight is my secret. That the means I see right now, what is outside as well as what is inside, isn't genuine, it is a device utilized to show me that my understanding is everything. That the way I saw points yesterday is the past. I request for assistance on what I am implied to absolutely see tomorrow. I use myself congratulations on having actually made it through one more round of life's everyday challenges with renewed stamina and gratitude for all I am doing to recover as well as enjoy.

I I see to it to do my ears and also squeeze my earlobes. I state caring features of exactly how thankful I am to have the present of hearing and also touch. Exactly how nice it is to have such a beautiful face as well as body, capable of terrific expression as well as inflammation. With simply a change of my features or a movement of my limbs, I can communicate to the people I like just how much they indicate to me, and also how much I like them. I search in the mirror as well as deal myself the very same affection. I smile and press.

I move in circles over my heart and joints as well as in lengthy lines down my limbs. I do the bottoms of my feet in fast backward and forward rhythms, pressing and pushing wherever it really feels finest. I check out the affirmations on my mirror as well as advise myself of all my body does that is right and also automatic, and wonderfully healthy and balanced. I assure it that I am taking great care of it and relief is taking place currently.

This is a time of deep nurturing. The power of touch is unmatched when it concerns producing a sense of relaxation. While I don't typically venture out for a massage, I make certain I provide myself a massage therapy on a daily basis.

When I'm done, I set, or I rest for a moment or 2 as well as let the oil saturate into my skin.

Temperature Guideline

Then I step into the shower as well as deal with my typical series of tasks under warm water. I do not utilize a great deal of soap, but make certain to make use of all-natural items (skin is an organ, exterior is inside). The oil on my skin enhances the lather of the majority of soaps, so much less is required. Then, I completed with a cool shower, as cool as I can stand it, and I take a minimum of two minutes however preferably concerning seven. I set a timer if required or listen to two or 3 songs. The very first few seconds under chilly water, I dance like a reward competitor in my corner, gearing up for the obstacle to find. As soon as I have actually got a grip on the rhythm of my breath as well as allow it go, I duck under the water and begin with my head. I let it get really cool. I enable the water rainfall over my face. I pinch my nose and also pointer back so I can massage therapy my eyes. With any luck, your shower head offers a consistent however gentle stream-- if it's shooting daggers, then this isn't mosting likely to really feel as good.

Consider swapping out shower heads, as I have actually found this part to be worth it! The chilly water brings swelling down, and I make sure you can visualize exactly how excellent it feels to muscles that are swollen, strained and pressed, and constrained by additive tissue that has actually accumulated in the orbital. This chilly shower can also be performed in the early morning as part of your everyday G.R.A.V.E.S. I've found it makes placing on make-up much easier if my eyes aren't as inflamed.

When my face gets extremely chilly, I relocate the water down to my thyroid at the base of my throat. In no way do you wish to produce pressure, hostility, or compression in this field. After the water brings my core temperature down in my breast and also over my body organs and stubborn belly, I turn around as well as do my back. I target my neck as well as shoulders.

I ensure to get my main body temperature level down and then target significant muscular tissue teams and also get them wonderful as well as cool also. The only thing I make certain of during this process, is not obtaining my head damp once more as it can launch a hypothermic feedback. So maintain the water neck down afterwards first minute.

As I mentioned, occasionally it aids if I place some music on or set a timer. While some days it is a difficulty to end up every shower by doing this, I locate that the result makes me feel incredible and the wellness benefits are amazing. Temperature guideline is a vital feature of the thyroid, and also in offering my body a reminder of what it seems like to cool down, I recognize I'm enhancing temperature regulation for the rest of my life. I learned this trick from listening to females with menopause deal with hot flashes, and professional athletes regulate metabolic function.

These 7 minutes showers are particularly practical right before bed, because they aid me to avoid severe evening sweats and also launch a more relaxed rest.

Eight Hours

Also my daughter, who is just about to turn 5, suches as to complete her shower with a cold blast. I'm leading by example below as well as wishing to establish a few daily behaviors into a rhythm that becomes something she can go back to time and again in her life.

I likewise take a lot of my cues from her. I go to bed with her every night at the exact same time, around 8pm. We read a few publications, set a reflection to play, and also we are typically sleeping by 8:30 -9 pm. Despite the fact that I'm fairly specific going to bed at 8pm and getting up at 4:20 am marks me as some kind of premature elderly person, I stick to these hrs as typically as possible. At the very most recent I attempt to be sleeping by 10pm. In between the hours of 10-2am every one of the organs in the body repair work themselves, so if I am burning the midnight oil, I am not enabling my system to repair itself. Instead, I am creating a situation of dis-ease.

Sparrow had problem with these hours. When we first fulfilled she would certainly awaken at 2:30 am frequently in a full sweat, not able to get back to sleep. Once we adjusted her rest routine, included a chilly shower prior to bed, set her do not interrupt hours, as well as determined that she would not grab the phone to examine the time in the middle of the evening, points boosted. Before interacting, when she would certainly awaken at 2:30 am, she would certainly search her phone for some useless Podcast or reveal on Netflix to assist her drop off to sleep once again.

What she stated made a difference in damaging this behavior for her was something I said throughout one of our sessions together. I asked that next time she woke up at 2:30 am, she just pick to not pick up her phone. That she just remain in bed, roll onto her back and offer herself approval to rest, to drop back asleep. As soon as she integrated the cold showers into this formula, her sleep problems significantly decreased.

Heaven light associated with computer system displays and so forth is really challenging on your body clock. I stay clear of checking out them 2 hrs before bed, or if I need to, I put on a pair of Blue Technology lenses (Google that with your postal code to locate an optometrist that brings them). I chose initially to obtain a pair over the counter since my prescription kept altering as my eye altered. I additionally had actually the included advantage of having had Lasik years prior to any type of thyroid eye illness manifested so my prescription wasn't extreme to start with. Working together with your eye doctor below will obtain you the assistance you need to make computer system work less of a pressure on your eyes during the day. I can not state what a difference this made for me during the hardest part of my Thyroid Eye Illness adventure.

The largest favor you ca do on your own if you fight with your eyes, is to prevent taking a look at a computer system in the evening. Pursue daytime hrs, or use a filter on your display for nighttime.

Enchanting Thyroid Eye Illness.

Allow's discuss this component of things for a min. The eyes are the hardest part of all of this to browse at times due to the fact that not seeing clearly can stop you in your tracks.

It was irritation in my eye, and also swelling that didn't go away, which clued me right into the truth that my thyroid might be at the heart of what was taking place for me. I have actually regarded my ideal eye as my inform since. The method it changed and altered, a lot to my dismay, made the indisputable truth of what was taking place inside me all the more apparent.

It was particularly difficult in the beginning, due to the fact that all I could see when I searched in the mirror was my eye. Even after three surgical procedures on my attractive eye, my "altered" eye is still occasionally all I can see when I search in the mirror.

Evidently, it is extra usual for TED clients to experience signs of dryness, eyelid retraction, tightness, and outcropping in both eyes. I have to admit, there were times when I wished both of my eyes would have been affected, so I might have looked rather in proportion. Having just one eye out of order made me feel like that timeless character in an old film that has a humpback and also one eye extending in a frightening method.

She is a sorceress or a witch. Someone every person hesitates of, capable of seeing things as well as doing evil magic.

As well as here is the thing: with every modification in the position of my eye came a change in perspective. My sight was physically transforming so that I would be forced to check out life in a new method. For two strong years I had problem with double vision, severe light level of sensitivity, and a failure to concentrate that was so disorienting I could not drive an automobile. For the initial three years of my little girl's life, I might not really see what she resembled unless I shut one eye. Had to depend on other senses to browse her treatment as well as our relationship. I think that handicap is responsible for our present capability to attach without needing to be in the exact same room. I don't depend on what I see outside, I review what I really feel inside to take care of her.

This instructed me the relevance of reviewing what I really feel on the inside in order to care for me.

The important things about Thyroid Eye Condition, is that before any type of repair or significant relief can be administered, the modifications have to have actually stabilized for a minimum of a year. When I heard this news, I was squashed. I wanted to look in the mirror and see myself again. I asked yourself if that would ever before occur. I made use of to fear mosting likely to the eye doctor, not desiring him to tell me what I believed to hold true: that points were getting worse, not better. Up till that conference with my endocrinologist when I made a decision to heal myself, I seemed like a passive victim of a condition wrecking my body.

As my eye stuck out further as well as even more out of its socket, and my eyelid retracted more and more, I grew weary of squinting and tired of sleeping with one eye open all the time. It just would not relax totally. Even in the evening with a mask over my eyes, my appropriate eye would not shut completely. I 'd awaken with it being so dry and swollen it would certainly take at the very least a hr to be able to kind of emphasis.

I have blue eyes. They are extremely light as well as somewhat special in color. When I was little bit, grownups made use of to talk about them at all times. I bear in mind really feeling annoyed due to the fact that the shade of my eyes was something I had no control over. I really did not think I was responsible for exactly how pretty they are. However this whole experience has actually educated me that I are accountable for their elegance, I are in charge of the means they provide themselves. I are in charge of what they express. I can let love shine from within as well as brighten the globe without, or I can allow frustration, temper as well as irritability brew. I can come to be that freaky looking character, unable of the world seeing plainly, worried to focus when she looks within.

Looking internal this way frightened me. I wouldn't have done it if I had not been so nauseous constantly looking without. I needed tranquility and also calm. When I opened my eyes, everything relocated and swam, edges were obscured, room merged. I couldn't recognize people in my life until they were within a few feet of me. Individuals began to read me as cold due to the fact that I simply really did not see them all right to greet. I started to take out. I went inside as well as remained.

As soon as I saw what was really there, I obtained caught up. I became aware of all of the flammable material I had collected that was littering the rooms of my house, my mind and also heart. That fire raving on the within not just had combustible debris in the kind of physical info, yet it was loaded to the gills with flammable particles I could not see, however that I recognized was lining the corridors of my values and also beliefs. I can see clearly that my thoughts and feelings resembled a whirlwind, fanning the fires to offensive elevations.

Chapter 7.

Chapter 6: Clearing the Debris You Can Not See.

Detoxing the Mind.

Equally as toxic substances build up in the physical body, toxic substances develop in ideas and sensations as well, contributing to a whipping wind that compels that fire better out of control.

Right around the very same time that I began to make adjustments to my diet and also lifestyle, my hubby and daughter and also I moved from Colorado to The golden state. We evacuated an area we had actually lived for over fifteen years, said goodbye to all of our family and friends, as well as went to Los Angeles. 8 months later, I brought my child back to Colorado on a two week trip for my parent's 45th wedding celebration anniversary and my secondary school reunion.

It took me 8 months to return to California.

Just to be clear on the timing, at this point I had been in remission with normal levels for two months. In the first 2 weeks of remainder I had at my parents' residence, I went through a psychological detoxification. I've pertained to describe those two weeks as psychological rehab. I involved see that my life was not a clear expression of my worths as well as beliefs. Initially I couldn't also see what I did worth as well as think. No pun in high gear vision, yet geez, it felt like there were two realities taking place-- the one within and the one without. The truth that others could see as real for me, as well as the truth that I viewed as true for myself.

Things had gotten so muddled as well as confused. What I understood to be true was that while I still loved my hubby as well as partner of over seventeen years, we can no more stay wed. We had actually produced an unhealthy dynamic because relationship, as well as I had to shift the ideas and also feelings I had there. I began to journal. I took notes during all of my telephone call with my hubby, and during the minutes of reflection I had each day. When I made the effort to look back over that conclusion of thoughts as well as feelings, I started to assemble the aspects I wished to maintain and also those that needed to be launched.

I intended to continue to be good friends with my soon to be ex-husband. I desired our daughter to experience the very best components of our relationship, and to moms and dad in a manner that was comprehensive of my partner's new partner. This was a very attempting time, as well as even as I place the words down in black and white here, I seem like there is this large elephant in the space that I am still frightened to discuss since I do not intend to be labeled or judged or determined as that individual. Yet I'm never going to get past the worry I really felt after that, if I don't own it currently.

So below it goes:.

I was an almost forty year old female that had actually been together with one male because she was twenty-one. I never assumed I 'd get separated, I never ever assumed I 'd have a child and 3 years later on leave my marriage. I never ever believed my partner would certainly find another female and also fall in love. I never thought he 'd seem like I was so vulnerable that he could not birth to inform me he 'd outgrown me for worry that it would be the final stroke and damage me. I never assumed I 'd need to reside in my parent's cellar with my child as well as scrape with each other a fresh start.

All of these information culminate right into a particular worry: that I am insufficient on my own. Insufficient to captivate a male forever, not enough to parent separately and also together with an overall complete stranger, not nearly enough to make a life on my own, insufficient to attract individuals I intend to collaborate with, insufficient to located an organization assisting individuals into genuine expression, insufficient period. Not enough. Not deserving enough of love and support from my household and my tribe.

That is an extensive concern, and it still rears it's awful head whenever I lose sight of my primary goal in life: to enjoy flat-out and emerge keeping that message.

I say that line so conveniently now, so simply, but it took three years of discussing my soul's purpose for me to do just that ... to place it out there in a such a details means. To possess that I am enough, present moment, to lead by instance and also beam my light.

Defying social convention and also loving my husband and his girlfriend right into a delighted place following among one of the most extensive experiences of viewed betrayal I have actually ever gone through, was challenging, however, for me there was nothing else selection.

I may be sometimes a sergeant when it comes to moderating my own habits and also relegating my choices, however when it comes to transforming the eyes of justice on my buddy, I simply can not see anything that needs judgment. Do not get me incorrect, I was unbelievably baffled and disoriented by my experience, however I likewise never ever leave what is stunning and also excellent. I could not embrace the despair. I learned that love does not ever pass away, and satisfied endings look various for everybody.

Throughout this whole procedure, I kept my diet regimen and also my new way of living routines even more intensely. I assume having to do this while coping with my moms and dads, obtaining separated, and also parenting under their roof covering was perhaps among the hardest points I have actually ever achieved in my life.

I got actual with the dark, and also I found that Thyroid Eye Condition made obtaining actual less complicated. It revealed me a clearer method to see.

Now, that is bat shit crazy.

Woo-Woo Town.

So yeah, looking outside myself really did not bring me tranquility. It made me wish to regurgitate. I simply flat out couldn't concentrate. I would certainly overlook at my sleeping infant and also see 4 eyes where there ought to just be two. I 'd seek to walk down a flight of stairs, as well as find my foot sensation for the side of a stair understanding I had no depth assumption whatsoever. I might no longer browse the world according to what had worked before.

I needed to obtain creative, and find new means of seeing all right to care for my lady, hold a job, as well as make a couple of significant life shifts.

I located those brand-new ways of seeing to originate from within. It was not easy at first, given that when I shut my eyes, all I might really feel was a whirl of stressed ideas manifesting as waves of stress and anxiety and also incapacitating muscle mass weak point. At first, I didn't intend to obtain still enough to truly have a look at what entered into developing those feelings of disease.

What I experienced originally, was akin to an experience I had throughout a few of my very early alpinism days. I once took place a twenty-one day backpacking trip. It was a guided trip, luckily, because one evening, at the end of a nineteen mile day, we discovered ourselves traversing a knife edge ridge in between two twelve thousand foot tops. I really felt upset at having actually been lead to do something so harmful at the end of a lengthy day. I really felt betrayed by my overviews, and distressed that they would conserve something so technological for the eleventh hour when we were so worn out. There had not been even sufficient area on the ridge for two of my feet side by side. As I hiked with the snow and began to go across the saddle, I purposely removed the climbing panic I felt by focusing on my actions, putting one foot securely before the other. I maintained my eighty pound backpack right over my hips as well as looked in advance concentrated through the blinding snow. There was absolutely nothing on either side of me to keep, nothing to lean against for safety. Just me, my equilibrium, as well as my sense of what was right. I relocated so rapidly throughout that saddle that I barely registered the experience. When I reached the opposite, I no longer felt panic, I really felt excitement, I was secure, and also in fact desired I would have taken pleasure in the going across extra. Gone was the anxiety as well as its area was eagerness for the following event.

Something type of comparable happened when I looked within for advice on browsing my life without. Inside, it felt dangerous, perilous, and negligent. I was worn out as well as day-to-day live was intimidating. It felt like there wasn't adequate space for me, as well as I was being pressed off balance by whipping winds.

It felt like I required to hurry and also simply obtain this going across over with, make it through this stretch of life. I intended to just instantaneously have the ability to look throughout the trip as well as see my destination beyond, clear as day.

Inside my ideas were lightening fast, generating emotions and experiences, stimulating reactions and repeatings quickly. Envision that quantity of activity inside a house on fire. Whipping wind, debilitating feelings, life on the side of control..

Soul's Purpose

I just said, "It felt like I needed to hurry and just get this crossing over with, get through this stretch of life. I wanted to just instantly be able to look across the journey and see my destination on the other side, clear as day."

And believe I'll be okay.

I have struggled with this word "believe." It once sounded too similar to words like trust, faith, know, and intuit. I felt like I could have faith on behalf of other people without hesitation, trust and intuit it would all work out for them, but when it came to me, I doubted. I didn't believe that faith would lead me on to the fulfillment of my desires.

How about that. I doubted, and the universe promptly drop kicked me into awareness. I needed a catalyst on my soul's path.

What I have come to understand, is this internal conflict has to do with living a life without purpose. I was not implementing my soul's purpose. Hell, I didn't even really have my soul's purpose pinned down. I just knew a few things about myself that were slowly dying as I did for others what I wouldn't do for myself. In my heart I knew this to be true:

1. I'm a good teacher.
2. I like connecting with people and helping them help themselves.
3. I enjoy interacting on a soul to soul level in a sacred space.
4. I love, love, love to write fiction.

This felt like a pretty broad base for defining my soul's purpose, and it wasn't news to me. What I couldn't wrap my mind around was what I was meant to make of these things. Naturally, being all hippy-dippy, I turned to astrology and numerology. I'm an ancient art historian by education and have an affinity for prehistoric Bronze Age civilizations in the Mediterranean. These maritime experts were some of the earliest people to map the heavens for navigation and chronological purposes. Astrology and numerology are to me like ancient mapping systems for potential navigation.

I've dabbled in having birth charts drawn up on occasion for my birthday, but hadn't ever had a one-on-one reading with what I'd consider an expert until the winter I divorced my husband. My friends, Gregory Paul Martin and his wife Cherie, gifted me with a heavily discounted short reading. It initiated a deep dive into certain aspects of my chart, particularly my rising sign.

I spent some time looking there and digesting what it meant to be a Leo rising with Saturn in the ascendant. I'm not even sure I'm explaining that accurately, but when I think about what it means, I see an old man in a straight jacket, forced to participate in a beauty contest. His talent is comedy, and his job is to make the audience laugh. That's my soul's purpose: get out there on that stage. Just get it out there. Break out like a sprout into the light and have a good time. Play a little in the sun. I was born under a crescent moon, and I'm certain that in the midst of Los Angeles--this glamorous little town, it feels safe to emerge with a message of Big Love.

It is strange to take comfort knowing what I am here to do is be uncomfortable.

When I began to look at things from this perspective, it became easier to be with friends and family as I made dramatic changes to my life. Answering their questions and regarding their opinions without becoming angry or defensive was and continues to be a daily exercise.

These discomforts are the debris, the flammable debris that wild wind whips into burning flames. At times in my life, I can watch it happen. I'll have an experience in a circumstance and think a thought and immediately feel a rotten feeling. It will evoke a reaction that reinforces that circumstance, and I'm locked in tight once again.

For example, let's say I have an experience with authority that makes me want to hide and avoid any sort of notice what so ever. I'll start to think thoughts about how uncomfortable I am being noticed, then I'll retreat to the point of stumbling and draw the focus of an entire room. Fear and confusion handicaps me.

That straight jacket is so comfortable!!!

I think I was raised in part to feel a degree of comfort in fear. The only trouble with this is, fear causes me disease. Fear is what I have used to motivate me most of my life. Fear of failure led to over preparation. Fear of poverty led to overworking and underpayment. Fear of abandonment led to hiding in someone else's shadow.

Now that I'm on my own, there is no where to hide. Moreover, I've got a witness. My little girl is here as the voice of love reminding me that being front and center on the stage is a beautiful place to be. She likes it best when I am goofy and odd, not when I am frustrated and dark. She likes to see that old man dance in a sparkly bikini wearing heels and making fun happen.

Knowing what I know now, doesn't make it any easier at times to avoid slipping into my shadow self. What it does do is make it easier to step back into the light. I'm jumping ahead a little bit. Let me get back to the magic. Let me remind myself what I did to release myself from the straight jacket of fear so I can dance with my little girl.

Born Again in Phillip Dixon's Pool

Right before I left California for Colorado, I met a shaman, a modern day near extra-terrestrial guru in Venice. I loved him at first sight.

I was on an adventure with a girlfriend. I had lived in LA for eight months, and had barely gone out or done anything social, mostly because I was seeing double, paranoid and freaked out chemically, and also because I felt like I looked weird. My friend cloaked our adventure in work, and took me to meet a well-known photographer.

Over his tequila at eleven in the morning, my new friend, Philip Dixon, called me out on my whole spiritual deal.

We had been introduced about a half an hour prior, and in that close window of time, he saw right through me. I saw the inside of his home, his sacred space, and he read my heart through my face. A Chinese teacher had shown him how to do it once, and there was no denying that the things he said were true.

Now upon accepting the invitation to meet him, this mystic mama with small town ways, raising her girl in the little big city of Lost Angels had no idea what to expect. I always say I'm not the type to do internet research on someone. Actions speak louder than words, and I like to have my own first impression and go from there. So apart from knowing he had photographed the first big supermodels in the 80s and 90s, I hadn't a clue about him. That fact alone had me wanting to bail, but my friend convinced me.

We pulled up outside of what appeared to be a cement bunker in a sort-of-okay part of Venice. A tall door stood ajar, and against it leaned a thin man in a dark smock. I flashed instantly to my favorite photograph of Gustav Klimt holding a cat. This guy's salt and pepper hair brushed his shoulders and the lines in his face were a mix of merry and mean, or wary, I couldn't decide. I followed him into the cool corridors of his home, and travelled back in time. I was somewhere in the Near East or on the shores of the Mediterranean perhaps 2500 years ago. Post and lintel construction in cement and wood, with stucco walls in pale cream made me feel at home. Instantly, I felt calm, the *wabi sabi* of the place did its trick, and when it unfolded into an open air courtyard with a pool and cacti in the middle, I felt my spirit inhale deeply for the first time in months. I was safe and inspired.

His home has been host to countless weddings, photoshoots, and classy events. I could tell that there was all this crazy energy passing through, but I couldn't feel any residue. His home flows, open throughout, and it can't be closed off from the elements, there are no screens in the windows, and just a few proper doors. Nevertheless it is a retreat, surrounded by a wall nearly twenty feet tall. It's a blend of rounded edges and hard surfaces, a lot like Philip's character.

Like his home he is spartan in communication and doesn't mince words. What he said to me over lunch that day felt solid. When he brushed my bangs off my face, titled my chin up towards the light and said to my friend, "See that?" I did not feel like a supermodel, I felt like a super freak!

My friend, the one who introduced us, knew exactly what he was pointing out.

I remember not moving, frozen under his observations. Then I retreated as he dropped his hand.

Let's keep in mind that Dixon has an editor's eye for the aberrant in the first place, and it is as though face reading is his dialect of the visual language. He's a photographer, really good with skin, sun, earth, sky and water. He has captured beautiful people in the simplest manner possible, an intoxicating blend of primitive and elegant. His work is sun soaked, mystic, and according to my vibe reader, very SoCal.

"*That*," he continued, "is about trauma." He sat back and waited for me to look up, then he went on. "Change your life, change your face."

The simplicity of it hit me like a ton of bricks.

I arrived in that moment, at the essential meaning behind my experience with Graves' Disease and Thyroid Eye Disease.

I didn't feel I was important enough to speak about what was in my heart, so the words died in my throat and poisoned my thyroid. After I had my little girl, all of those lost thoughts in my heart came out in such a rush I couldn't handle it. At the same time, it became super important that I see my situation differently, so the pressure from that need built up and changed the position of my right eye by materializing in scar tissue. Even though I could not see clearly, physically, for two years, I was turning inward and seeing my true self for the first time in perhaps my entire life.

It was in the middle of the turning inward that I found myself having lunch with Philip.

My friend relieved the awkward moment by mentioning that she'd like a dip in his pool. Philip consented. We walked back.

We arrived and made as if to skip the swim and just leave, but I excused myself to use the restroom. I took one look at my reflection in the mirror and I just wanted to shed my skin. I wanted to step out of me and be born again. I walked out of there and took off my dress, stripped to my panties, and stepped into the pool that ran uninhibited through his home like a river. I spent the next thirty minutes alone, under the open air in the center of his cement sanctuary. I kept my ears underwater, listening to the beat of my own heart. When I got out, I sunned myself on a stretch of concrete porch until I felt my skin turn a new color. Then I put on my clothes, embraced my unconventional healer, and cried in silent release the whole way home.

Since that day, I have acted at nearly every turn in a effort to change my life. To shape it in a way that is a full and authentic expression of my true self.

Chapter 8
Chapter 7: Reorienting and Bridging the Gap to Big Love

MMJ

I'm about to get clear and clean about something that I've hidden for years. Remember earlier, when I said I was burner? That I liked to burn the candle at both ends and the midnight oil? Well, ever since I started getting wicked migraines, I've also liked to burn doobie.

At moments in my life when I have taken a break from pot, or let my conditioned feelings of guilt and shame about using it medicinally get the better of me, that is when I can map out what I have come to understand as thyroid flares. Somehow, I knew enough at the age of nineteen to decide that no matter how bad my migraines became, I would never use a synthetic remedy or pain reliever. I had watched people in my life build up tolerances to these medications, and be consistently debilitated by both the pain of a migraine, and the hangover of its relief.

At about the same time that I started getting into yoga, I also began to make lifestyle and diet choices in line with what made me feel good physically. While I had friends and colleagues I knew turn to anxiety medications and alcohol, I turned to doobie and food. I became a vegetarian and went along my merry hippy way. By the time I made it to graduate school about three years later, I had found a great balance and what I knew to be an even keel. I had just enough fire to keep me energized and optimistic, but not enough stress to fan the flames into a frenzy.

But then I moved away from most of my family and my partner, and I got all weird once graduate school started. I figured I couldn't do the doobie thing and be a serious student at the same time. I started getting regular headaches and turning more and more to conventional medicine for relief. One day it occurred to me that I had taken ibuprofen every day for a week straight and beyond that. My headaches were patterned and predictable. I began altering the course of my day, getting up and running before school. I made time for me before I got down to business.

At that time I lived with my sister, and we were training for the Portland marathon. She used doobie recreationally, and I remember finally asking her for a little. I would have a little first thing in the morning, and then we would go run.

Pretty silly, huh? I was a graduate teaching fellow in ancient art history taking a full load of coursework plus four language classes a term. I graduated with above a 4.0 and wound up with a full ride to Columbia's PhD program. I did it all on a hit of doobie first thing in the morning.

I had no problem flying below the radar in graduate school, because I was very private and most of my fellow students were married. It didn't bother me so much, at that time, what other people might think if they found out. I was a responsible adult doing well in the world. I spent months traveling without it and fared really well, as long as I kept my stress levels down and rested a lot.

Then, when I got pregnant with my girl, I had a similar wave of doubt where I questioned whether I should continue to use doobie while pregnant. I did a lot of reading on the subject, but ultimately it wasn't science that influenced my decision, but rather what I perceived the expectations were of others. This was my tribal conditioning superseding my own knowledge of self.

I spent my first trimester wrestling with this decision. I know now that what was kicking on during that time was a thyroid flare, and I couldn't read it clearly because there was a lot of change going on inside my body. I had never been pregnant before, so some of what I was experiencing I chalked up to that. I didn't even think to address it with my midwife.

I made decisions during that first third of my pregnancy that had serious repercussions. This business of Graves' Disease is incredibly psychological, and I experienced first hand what Jessica Somerville Ruffolo and Robert A. Stern write about in their 2001 article "What is wrong with me? I'm not myself anymore." Published by the Graves' Disease and Thyroid Foundation, Inc..

It felt like my usual self, the one who was outgoing and happy to be with people and doing things, had shriveled into a frightened mouse, scared and incapable of moving for fear of being caught. I felt paralyzed, my heart racing, and this sensation only increased as my pregnancy progressed.

Knowing I could not turn to any sort of antidepressant or anxiety medication at this stage in my pregnancy, I went back to what I knew worked. The relief I felt immediately was incredible. I was preoccupied writing down all of the worries that consumed me while my baby grew inside me, and then, I stopped listing those worries and started listing the gifts.

I shifted from the mentality of fear and oppression, to one of heart-centered courage. I allowed that gentle nudge to blossom into a full bloom during meditation, and then I cultivated that sensation the rest of the day. I let the guilt and shame thoughts settle and disappear. I knew that the gift of peace within was worth fostering, and I began to look for ways to balance my lifestyle with this herb in a way that would carry me through motherhood.

It has been no small feat, and whenever I get low, (because yes, that still happens--it's called life and PMS, and we will talk about such obstacles later), I remind myself that there are responsible ways to go about medicating naturally. For example, I make sure that I have at least three hours between the time I medicate in the morning and when my daughter wakes up. I ensure that if there is an emergency (migraine or other surprise), that I have a responsible way to take care of myself. I keep edibles in appropriate places. I also don't lie to my little girl about this stuff. It doesn't feel good to lie to her about anything, so I am frank when I say that this is medication and I make it myself so I have just what I need when I need it and there is no room for error there.

Here is the thing: we follow a restricted diet, so it isn't easy to just walk into a dispensary and choose any old edible. They are loaded with sugars and grains and dairy or soy or nuts. Moreover, they take some getting used to, and dosages vary. I find I have greater accuracy and I'm capable of responding more accurately if I have made my own.

I keep it simple. I just make coconut oil. I use kief and a slow cooker designed for cheese dip at a party. I use a ratio of 1 gram of kief to 1 cup of oil. I put everything in there together and let it sit overnight.

I remember the first time I talked with a client about this. I was all hesitant to talk about pot with her because we have people in common and both of us are moms. Then right before the fourth of July, we got started talking about navigating holidays and special occasions (again more on this later), and the subject of alcohol came up.

Clearly alcohol is a big to be avoided in your first three months of making this change, and then only on occasion after that and in extreme moderation. It was my client who said, "I'm okay without alcohol, I don't like it that much, but I am thinking about getting into pot." So, I set aside our lesson for that day and took the opportunity to walk her through how I have found it to be immensely helpful and why.

Here is the basic breakdown of benefits and targeted symptoms:

1. A whole food nutrient
2. Anxiety and paranoia modulator
3. Depression and mood stabilizer
4. Appetite stimulant and digestive aid
5. Sleep regulator
6. Perspective adjustor

Perspective Adjustor

"What do you mean, exactly, by perspective adjustor?" my client asked.

I drew an analogy between ginkgo and pot. Some people take ginkgo because they believe it will enhance their memory, among other things. They pay attention and look for validation that it is, indeed, enhancing their memory, or no, it isn't. The same is true for this herbal supplement. It might not work for everyone, but it certainly works for me.

It brought immense relief from the physical pain and discomfort of the migraines that were a daily symptom of Thyroid Eye Disease. Sometimes the discomfort would be so bad, I remember feeling like I wanted to take an icepick to the inner corner of my right eye. I was sure it would provide just the relief I needed. Shove it in there, give it a little stir and voila, all that tension would dissipate. Given how violent that solution is, the alternative of pot seemed rather benign. It also brought levity to a very dark mental condition and emotional lack of well being. (Even just coming up with that ice pick solution for the problem speaks of how sincerely dark my mentality was at times!)

In light of darker thoughts on the horizon, I decided I'd forego the guilt and shame I associated with being a mom who preferred pot to wine. I vowed to be responsible for my little girl, and I make sure I am capable of responding 99% of the time. I am considerate about timing medication, and I stick to the minimum necessary as a general rule.

I've been asked before if I stuck to edibles or did I also smoke during the toughest parts of Thyroid Eye Disease. I'll answer this frankly because I know I would have really valued this information when I was researching. I consistently used edibles, but also vaped and smoked throughout the course of my illness (migraines and edibles do not mix well together if the timing is off--they can be hard to keep down--and vaping is immediate relief, but having that ready was a challenge on the go). I had the good fortune of being able to see first hand the effect pot had on my eyes, because I had one control, my unaffected eye, and one eye under siege. I documented the symptoms and effects of medication and determined my ideal course of action. Getting this down to a science was one of the most challenging but helpful things I did to bring myself into remission.

Coming to a place of acceptance about using this herb with such a social stigma, helped me resolve a deep internal conflict and experience peace. The thoughts I was thinking about it were a form for self-sabotage, and an excuse to feel guilt and shame, to perpetuate dis-ease. These thoughts and feelings began at a time when the laws and culture around pot were very different. It is so nice that now it is considered appropriate medication. The first time I received a MMJ card, it was for migraines associated with Graves' Disease, and the physician who wrote the script for me let me know I was definitely not alone. There were other Graves' patients medicating for migraines this way.

I took this shift from self-consciousness to self-acceptance, and that empowered me. I began to look at what was going on in my life from a different angle. I saw the decisions I was making as being increasingly in line with what I value and believe. I watched as one right action after another manifested when I kept my thoughts focused on love. I wanted love in my life, and for the people in my life to love one another. The key to my healing was to love the people and situations I once believed were unloveable.

This was a tall order I also asked of my family and friends. I asked them in one fell swoop to do three things: 1. To honor my decision to divorce my partner of seventeen years. 2. To have no judgment or ill words about what motivated our decision, especially in front of my daughter. 3. To honor my ex-husband's new partner as a member of our modern family.

I asked for help in making my life's changes and received a miracle. I practiced self-love, asked for love, and received Big Love.

Rainbows, Hearts and Unicorns

Before I knew about everything we just talked about, the diet and lifestyle factors that contributed to Graves' Disease, I had no idea what eating gluten and burning midnight oil was doing to my body physically. Implementing right action habits in these departments was concrete and within my visible control. I began to feel stronger physically, and could navigate overmedication and coming off of medication.

But, because my eye surgeon wouldn't consider orbital deconstruction, eyelid retraction repair, or the other elements of repairing my eye until it had gone a year with no changes, I knew I had at least that long to wait.

I also knew I had another year of looking the way I did, of seeing with double vision, of migraines, and eye strain. This was very challenging emotionally and intellectually, but it gave me the time I needed to start to see clearly patterns in my behavior. During that year, and the year that I went through surgery, one every four months, I saw these patterns with even greater clarity.

What I saw both surprised me, and humbled me.

While I had gained a grasp on my physical symptoms, and believed I was doing all that could be done there, I didn't yet believe I made the change energetically. I was still learning when it came to ingesting emotions and intelligence.

Life seemed so nuts at times and overwhelming. I felt like I was melting down from all of the research and information I had gathered. I had to stop looking up symptoms and remedies, supplements and products. I went on an information diet that also excluded current events and pop culture. I haven't owned a television since I lived with my parents in high school, so that wasn't an issue. What kept me down intellectually was the time I spent on the web and social media. I couldn't escape election news or popular opinion on any number of scary hot topics having to do with sex, children, abduction, racism, sexism, the list goes on and makes me ill. Literally. I can feel the pit of my stomach clench and my insides get scared.

That sensation is a red flag, and I've come to recognize the feeling and the thought that creates that feeling as not conducive to my good health. I don't ingest information like that anymore. Sure, when I confess about not knowing all of the latest tragedies, it doesn't always go over well with new friends. I'm considered socially irresponsible or negligent by some.

Nevertheless, I know that I'm in no way contributing to Big Love in the world if I resonate with fear, this is a legitimate reason not to be informed. I trust that the information I must know will arrive in time.

In the same way that I follow an information diet, I also follow an emotional diet. The combined approach is something I refer to as, "Rainbows, Hearts, and Unicorns." All I want to engage with comes down to one of three things: light, love, and miracles.

I recognize that the only way I can truly make the world a brighter place to be, is by influencing my immediate sphere--by shining my light so that I can see my way, and others might be better able to see theirs. If I think I am alone in a dark room, then I think, "Light up, it is within you to be bright." When I shine I can at least see the path before me and all that is illuminated by my beam of focused light and intention. If I connect to one other person who is also living from place where her heart light shines bright, then together, we are two lights in that room and everything is brighter. Get enough people together and the walls of that room disappear into light, love, and miracles. Change happens. We get brighter, for all to see, and bring lost souls home.

There have been challenges along the course of this emotional diet, and it is always interesting to see where they come up. Sometimes it is as simple as feeling vulnerable after posting to social media. Usually, I have recurring thought patterns that are initiated by interactions with authority and surround money. I know these things to be true, and as I have watched myself navigate challenges with healthcare and finances as a newly single mom, I have watched my thought patterns create emotions that led to feelings. I usually react in a predictable way, with fear or anxiety. Then I follow the model that I learned as a kid, "Hope for the best, but prepare for the worst." The tension rises from wondering how I am going to prepare, how will I manage it all, and as I wonder, and try to see how to make it happen, I can feel the muscles crank in tighter behind my right eye.

Every physical symptom I've experienced with Graves' Disease I can connect with an emotion and feeling that is inspired by a thought about a circumstance. The thoughts and feelings are usually anxious or fearful, they suggest a lack of control or authority over my health and choices. They disempower me, and divorce me from the truth, which is that love is the only real thing in this life. That Big Love, the one that makes my heartbeat on automatic, the one that fills my girl with laughter in her sleep, the Big Love that we share as family. There is no need to be afraid, to hold my eye open out of fear or to stare down the right action. There is no need for my heart to race with apprehension, for my muscles to grow weak and tremble. There is no need for me to break out into an endless sweat, to race in this experience of life. There is no need to worry.

There is no need for a thyroid flare, because I can choose love at any time.

Chapter 9
Chapter 8: The Big Obstacles

Identifying the Root of Fear

Finding the root of my fear is a work in progress. (Email me and I'll help you do this if you are struggling: heathermaerussell@gmail.com.) The thing that has been like a roadmap on the journey is what Carolyn Myss calls body scanning. It is a systematic energetic check-in with your body based on chakras. I combined the chakra body scan (email me for more on this) with the planets and houses in astrology to get a clearer picture of what is going on within. I approach each house like it is a room in my home, and then I scan the room for things to give away. I scan it on each chakra level. This work is at the heart of my transformation from being in a state of disease to transforming into a consistent condition of ease. It is about cleaning house of all the debris that is fuel for inflammatory thoughts and feelings.

Each chakra holds information on the ways in which we distract ourselves from experiencing inner peace in various areas of life. I was overwhelmed at first with the amount of work to be done, and I needed a path to follow. I started with an eight-week intensive and now, each month I focus on one house, four days per chakra. I write down what I discover in each place like an inventory. I exercise what needs to be expelled and shine light on what needs polishing. This is a consistent and recurring exercise, and at the heart of any coaching I do.

Graves' Disease is to me like an inner terrorist. It is the manifestation of many things, but for me in particular it started with my response to someone I know who bullied me as a kid, and more so as a young woman. I shoved and buried that experience so far down into my guts that it went to seed and sprouted. It sprawled like roots into plumbing and constricted the flow of energy below it. It shut me down at the third chakra, the seat of my self-confidence. It skewed my understanding of family and partnership.

Instead of breathing in and out of my heart chakra, I held my breath, I took on responsibility for all I loved and surrendered nothing. I never spoke my truth, or used my voice to share. I had lost sight of what I had to offer.

That now mythic bully keeps me small as an adult, ensuring that I feel alone and hide, that I am defenseless and subject to the whims of other people in a cruel world. It attacks me from within, goaded on by whatever fuel it can find. Extinguishing these rogue flames that leap when fanned by negative thoughts and feelings is an everyday challenge. There have been times during this whole journey that I have wanted to just lay down, face first on the floor and never get up. Times when it just seems easier to give up.

Seeing everything in double, incapable of negotiating streets in the dark, or stairs during the day, taught me that the reality I perceived on the outside wasn't really real. It was so clearly an illusion, made up of crossed beams of light and a miracle on the inside. It taught me not to put too much stock into what I thought I saw. Reaching for something that isn't there wasn't just a metaphor. That was real, I couldn't see the right glass to grab, I could only choose one over the other in my sight and pray nothing broke if I was wrong.

Isn't that a great metaphor for life? Nothing I saw was real, it was all in my mind. Nothing I thought I thought was real, it was all in the past. I had to start over and have faith that what was true would rise like cream to the surface and I would know it as such because it would taste sweet and rich, and feel like satin or velvet.

The whole task of navigating life with this new awareness has been too much to bear more times that I can count. My experience tells me I'm not alone in this, every woman I interviewed while writing this book said as much. There is no shame in feeling this way. There is no shame and there is no guilt, if I surrender to love and get back up. Just get back up. I tell myself whenever my throat tightens like a noose, to let go, surrender into Big Love and get up.

In this life, Big Love's got your back. Get up on that unicorn and slide down that rainbow into the open arms of all you love and all who love you.

Can I Handle the Seasons of My Life

Every time I hear *Landslide* and Stevie Nicks asks if she can handle the seasons of her life, I start to cry and sing along when she says, "Oh oh, I don't know."

Commitment is a funny thing. I have no problem with committing to external things, but committing internally to getting back on that unicorn every time and believing, is a way of being that requires more of an effort on occasion. Fear is the breaker of commitments and the forger of bad deals. It tries to persuade me to sell my unicorn.

That is really at the crux of all of this. This question of whether I am capable of handling all of life's transitions with grace still keeps me up at night. I find that I ask myself these kinds questions on a regular basis, so I mapped out when they come up and noticed a pattern:

1. Questions about health and sustaining remission: every month during PMS, mid summer.

2. Questions about relationships and Big Love: every month during PMS, anniversaries and birthdays.

3. Questions about abundance and security: every month during PMS, at the holidays and the new year.

4. Questions about self worth and career choices: every month during PMS, during the last few days of the month, right before the majority of bills are due.

Noticing a trend? Yep, PMS is the single biggest obstacle I face on a regular basis for maintaining good condition physically, mentally, and emotionally. I once explained to a guy friend of mine why this time of the month can be so hardcore. He just didn't get what the big deal is or what it is about it that makes some women go nuts. I told him to imagine that every month, something inside you that has the potential to become another heart beating and soul shining dies. Women experience expelling that potential and reinitiating the process over and over, again and again, about 450 times over the course of their life. For the sensitive type, this can almost be too much chemistry to bear, or too much physical effort to endure if imbalance is present.

The themes of loss, transformation, and transition are aligned with memories, and memories are often aligned with specific moments in time. Time is the keeper and time is also the healer. Once I made it through an entire year, practicing what works well for me, I had had the opportunity to navigate anniversaries that were emotionally challenging and come out on the other side in good health.

At first these were simple occasions, the holidays, and birthdays, and events. It isn't just that it is challenging to say no to the traditional fare my mom always makes when it comes to food, it is. But what is harder than saying no, is continuously saying no, because the people who love me the most are the most frequent to forget. Emotionally, I also have strong ties to their expectations, and until I let go of needing to fulfill their expectations it will continue to be hard for me.

I also have emotional reasons for preferring certain foods at certain times, and certain thoughts accompany these foods. Nipping these cycles in the bud from either angle works. Choosing one right move after another in line with my wellbeing is the only thing that consistently holds me accountable for healing from within.

I begin with the food because it is physical, then I move on to the content of conversation, and the emotions I choose to experience. One right choice, physically, emotionally, mentally, followed by another right choice leads to happiness. A Course in Miracles enlightened me on the true meaning of healing: "to heal is to make happy." It is that simple. Choose what makes you truly happy in body, mind, and soul.

The Significance of Others

Sometimes the choices we must make in alignment with our happiness are tough, and they mean that life will never be the same.

Our error is in assuming that "never be the same" means, "never as good as this." I wonder if a caterpillar thinks the same thing as it is weaving a cocoon and preparing for change. I doubt it. It is a cruel trick we play on ourselves, because we are here to learn and grow and change is the only constant and if we are focused on being happy and therefore healthy, then "never the same" means, "always the best or something better."

That face down on the floor, never going to get up feeling was the most intense when the central relationship in my life changed dramatically. It was like my compass needle had detached. I was disconnected from my guide for finding North, and I thought life without my husband would never be as good as life with him.

Whenever I visit Graves' Disease forums, I inevitably come across a post made by a husband, pining for his wife. He feels like Graves' Disease and Thyroid Eye Disease have stolen her, and in her place left an unimaginable person. Not his wife, not his friend, but an angry and defensive witch, mean to him and unforgiving. It breaks his heart because the woman he loves doesn't exist anymore.

He aches for the same person she aches to be again.

I often wonder if that is what my husband experienced. I do know that I offered him all of the hurt in my heart, and showed him all of the weak places in my soul. I offered up what I could not bear to carry any longer. He was my best friend, and I didn't know how to ask for more love. So instead, I just cracked open my pandora's box and out spilled my shadow side.

Until I recognized that it was for me to clear, that he could not rid me of my debris, I do believe I punished him for being free. I somehow made it seem selfish that he was healthy and pursuing his dream. It wasn't my intention, it was just that what was happening on the inside was so unbearable, and I had opened the door and let the fire out. It was genuinely horrifying to be so quick to get pissed, so easy to get exasperated. It was even more horrifying to look in the mirror and see a physical manifestation of those emotions.

What was going on in my life that needed my undivided attention and a condition of panic for me to address it? The attitude of a patient with hyperthyroid is intense, and traveling through some of the forums and groups can really be scary at times. Graves' Rage is real, and definitely a veiled cry for Big Love. I was ugliest to my husband because he loved me unconditionally.

He was smart enough to continue growing while I re-calibrated.

My astrological chart also indicates that one of this life's learning grounds for me is that of relationships and shared resources and responsibilities. I had not addressed aspects that were out of balance in this area of my life, and so naturally, it collapsed.

I did a great job of clearing the debris and watching a phoenix fly from the ashes.

My next challenge here is to learn to do all of this again. To be that contestant and get out on that stage and share my message. To feel attractive and feel like sharing. To accept invitations and call people back. To follow through on all things, including my best intentions. These are the things that keep my relationships in balance, and welcome new relationships in.

My desire to be social is closely tied to my thermometer. If I get hot flashes at the thought of meeting friends on my night off, or saying yes to a date, then I know there is something I'm not addressing on an emotional and spiritual level. Over the course of the last year, I have made a very determined effort to iron out and write down places where I have energetic blocks and obstacles when it comes to communication and fulfilling my soul's purpose.

The result has been beyond expectation and according to my deepest desires. I divorced my husband and that day wrote a list of what I loved so much about him. Then I wrote a list of what I most desired in my future partner. He showed up within two months. I wrote a go-time to transition from one job that brought stress, to another that brought greater independence and stability. Less then five months later it happened. I declared I wanted to write my Graves' Disease story about what worked for me and help other people help themselves, and I finished the manuscript eight months later. I set a goal to publish three books this year and I am on target.

These are all miracles. These are all things that have incrementally saved my life. Finding my purpose and aligning my everyday with it has made all the difference. Knowing that my mission is to love in a very big way and get that message across in writing, is all I need to live a life on purpose and with great happiness. To heal is to make happy.

Relationships are a source of great happiness if we choose them wisely.

These are where we get the nutrients we need emotionally. In the same way that you watch what you eat and take in informationally, it is also important to watch what you take in emotionally. Systematically ridding your life of toxic relationship dynamics is essential to good happiness. Sometimes this means divorcing friends or family members, and it doesn't have to be a spouse.

I needed the benefit of a detox period away in order to feel my most important relationships out. And I mean that. I didn't try to "see" them for what they were. Seeing was hard. I relied on other senses to guide me. I focused on how they felt, what taste they left in my mouth, what thoughts I heard in my head, and whether something smelled foul. Then I made decisions and stuck to them. I wrote everything down so I would know where I was when emotionally.

These journals are a touchstone for me, and I am so grateful I have accounts of wise choices and intentions.

Big Self Love

"You are as much of a power magnet in your life as the things and people that are most important to you. Please, invest in yourself as such."

This is an affirmation I need to read every day, so I can remind myself that I am setting an example for my daughter. She is learning from me about how to take care of herself so she can serve others. It might be a device I use to keep me motivated and choosing right action, right thoughts, right feelings in line with my well being, but it is a powerful device. Naturally, I wouldn't wish this experience on her, but I am aware she will have her own experiences of adversity to navigate, and part of my responsibility as a parent is to model useful skills for that.

What I do know, is that my daughter was a catalyst in life that I am forever grateful for. It is my most important relationship, and one of my biggest sources of happiness and good health. She has given me the perspective of love.

Why deny that we are among a unique group of people? We are those who have seen double for a sustained period of time in life, and still we have carried on doing what we do! What an amazing accomplishment! Again, the women I've interviewed for this book are living accomplished lives and doing amazing things in spite of living with Graves' Disease. They are raising families, holding together careers and marriages. Typical superhero stuff.

I recently had the fantastic experience of taking my daughter to story time at our local library. Kids are so awesome at calling it like they see it. This little four-year-old girl took one look at me and straight-up asked, "How come your eyes are like that?"

I swallowed hard around a lump of emotion in my throat. I know I look way more normal and feel a lot better than I have in years, but still this comment cut to the quick. I took a deep breath and replied, "My eyes are special and unique so that I can see all that I am meant to see in this life. Isn't that amazing?"

"Yes," she replied, clearly impressed.

In that moment, I once again had confirmation that I am developing a superpower of unique perception. It is the ability to hear my Higher Self asking me to see love, Big Love--Big Self Love, as the only real thing. It is a felt sense. It is cool peace of mind, and a refreshed and humbled heart. It is a light that cannot be dimmed but is steady, constant, and undeniable.

Why then do I deny it? Why do I banish it to the corners of my mind?

This is the game of yin yang, right wrong, peace war, hope worry, fear love. If I recreate by dwelling in past experiences of negativity, then I am banishing love to the corner.

Boom. Point for Graves' Disease!

What if I choose instead to shift, to choose wisely more often than not in the direction of love? This is the experiment, this is where true alignment happens. This is what remission is all about.

There are patients for whom remission happens, and then it stops happening. This, I believe, is at the root of the reason why disease ebbs and flows. Our thoughts are at times negative and at others positive. How smoothly we transition back and return to center, to Big Love, determines the quality of our daily life. It determines our health.

Spontaneous, or quantum, healing happens after a shift in awareness from self-consciousness to self acceptance. This is a daily practice for me, and the most important thing I do for my wellbeing.

Heart to heart, this is the most important part of this book. Daily I make a practice of accepting that the past has no meaning. Only today and all it offers has the meaning I assign it.

I prescribe good health every day, and practice it.

Chapter 10
Conclusion: Future Tools

The Next Right Step

Now that I know how the full spectrum of thyroid imbalance feels, I am a lot clearer about reading my levels without the help of blood work. I have mapped the course of symptoms and life circumstances and can recognize the patterns created by my responses to what I digest physically, mentally, and emotionally. The pattern began in college and it took almost twenty years and nearly dying or going blind for me to see how it all fit together like a puzzle. Now that I know how important it is to be spiritually aligned and in a place of happiness, it makes it that much easier to get back into balance when I feel things slipping.

So here is my simple Big Self Love formula for living with these diseases:

1. Make what I eat be an act of peace not war: AIP Paleo based approach to this and any supplements.

2. Make what I feel be about happiness more often than not: to heal is to make happy so I nature bathe, massage, take salt baths, laugh and do yoga every day.

3. Make what I think be about cultivating inner peace: practice mental discipline in the form of information dieting, meditation, and journaling to release any attack thoughts.

I have learned that diet is the easy part, and sticking to it is one of the best things you can do to turn that cruise ship around. Diet alone, unfortunately, isn't enough. Autoimmune diseases are the manifestation of inner conflict. They are what happens when our actions are not in line with what we value and believe. It can be as simple as having the wrong job, or staying in friendships and relationships that do not serve you and by extension the greater good. Making life changes that bring about spiritual transformation is what Graves' Disease and especially Thyroid Eye Disease call for. They force us to readjust our understanding of time and space. Our hearts and minds race, and our eyes see double. We have complicated some aspect of life that needs to slow down and become unified. In my experience that aspect is spiritual and unique to each soul in the midst of their experience.

I found myself wanting to go within, to know my soul better, and seek an understanding of why and how this had all happened. This exploration led me to A Course in Miracles, and there, in workbook exercise number twenty, I quickly found my mantra: "I am determined to see."

At first I didn't know what that meant, but I knew it was meant for me.

I quickly learned that it meant I am determined to see that I am cared for, held tenderly, and celebrated as a soul here to fulfill its purpose. I studied my astrological chart, numerology, and energy centers and found my path to be about emerging with a message. That message is one of Big Love and I write to spread my message.

If there is some part of you that is confused, putting your finger on it now, I believe, helps healing happen faster. Deepak Chopra reminds us that a shift in awareness, an awakening, a return to love is required for healing to happen.

And it happens.

It happens again and again, every day. It is a choice. Marianne Williamson, author of Return to Love, talks about the only drama in life being the one where we walk away from love and then return to love. All drama can be brought back to this one basic move.

Move in the direction of love, Big Love, Big Self Love. Use your mind to walk you back there each time you feel you thoughts and feelings go astray. This journey is cyclical and we will be given the opportunities again and again to make this choice between Love and Fear. Perhaps this is why some of us experience recurring episodes or moments when thyroid imbalance comes back, stronger than before. Medication will placate, but the underlying energy that is in conflict will make itself heard eventually. This is why autoimmune diseases cluster and change shape. If at first we don't answer the call, our soul's shout to be heard that we are off course, it will try another avenue.

If this sounds too abstract, then sit with it for a moment and consider if your discomfort is something you can live with. Consider whether you feel safe knowing "experts" say you will have this dis-ease for the rest of your life. Do you have peace in your heart knowing you might not ever know what life off of medication feels like? Do you sleep well at night knowing you are doing all you can to be sure your other eye doesn't suffer, or worse yet, both eyes have a relapse?

If you are okay with these things, if you can live with a part of you subscribing to these options as reality, then fantastic, continue on, and love be with you.

If there is a part of you that can't accept what I just said, a part that doesn't feel content with the idea that this current version of you might be the you from here on out, or the you until your levels change or stress ensues and you react with a flare according to the way you imagine you will, then let's get down to it. Get down to the business of decoding where this inner conflict begins and resolve it. (If you are determined to see, mail me at heathermaerussell@gmail.com and we will do a quick tarot card pull to get a clearer picture.)

I have spoken with women who have completely curtailed their lives and curtained off their families because they are incapacitated by these diseases, and my heart just aches for them. It is a lonely and cold place to be when we isolate and go dark. There are so many ways to step out of the dark and into the light but it's easy to forget that in the thick of it.

Some of us will turn to a life of faith and a practice of inner peace, some to the trusted confidence of counselors, some to the encouragement and forward thinking of wellness coaches. Whatever your path is to unity and inner calm, find it and take it. Invest in yourself, for the good of all. You can do it, and this work will likely be the most important mission of your life.

Lead by example for the people you love, and take good care of yourself so that you can live a life of happiness and good health. Remission is a beautiful place to be, and beautiful things, people, and experiences gather here.

www.ingramcontent.com/pod-product-compliance
Lightning Source LLC
LaVergne TN
LVHW041231150826
845673LV00008B/2354

* 9 7 9 8 7 5 8 8 7 5 3 9 1 *